WOMEN'S HEALTH— MISSING FROM U.S. MEDICINE

RACE, GENDER, AND SCIENCE
Anne Fausto-Sterling, General Editor

Titles published in the series:

Feminism and Science (1989)
Nancy Tuana, Editor

The "Racial" Economy of Science:
Toward a Democratic Future (1993)
Sandra Harding, Editor

The Less Noble Sex:
Scientific, Religious, and Philosophical
Conceptions of Woman's Nature (1993)
Nancy Tuana

Love, Power and Knowledge:
Towards a Feminist Transformation of the Sciences (1994)
Hilary Rose

Women's Health–
Missing
from U.S. Medicine

Sue V. Rosser

Indiana University Press

BLOOMINGTON AND INDIANAPOLIS

The paper used in this publication meets the minimum requirements of American
National Standard for Information Sciences—Permanence of Paper for Printed
Library Materials, ANSI Z39.48-1984.

∞™

Manufactured in the United States of America

Library of Congress Cataloging-in-Publication Data
Rosser, Sue Vilhauer.
Women's health—missing from U.S. medicine / Sue V. Rosser.
p. cm. — (Race, gender, and science)
Includes bibliographical references and index.
ISBN 0-253-34991-5 — ISBN 0-253-20924-2 (pbk.)
1. Sexism in medicine—United States. 2. Medicine—Study and teaching—
United States. I. Title. II. Series.
RA564.85.R67   1994
610'.82—dc20   94-9745

1 2 3 4 5 00 99 98 97 96 95 94

CONTENTS

Acknowledgments

The ideas, theories, and examples that form the foundation of this book came from developmental phases in my education, interdisciplinary seminars, and lectures, as well as chance encounters and passing conversations with colleagues and friends. These individuals contributed to the evolution of my thoughts in abstract and complex ways, too difficult to enumerate.

My family, Charlotte, Meagan, and Caitlin, and the Women's Studies staff, Linda, Judith, and Amy, supported me and the book in concrete ways that permitted it to be translated from ideas into reality. The suggestions of my colleague Thavolia Glymph provided very useful insights for chapter 6. I am especially grateful to Charlotte Hogsett for reading and editing numerous drafts of the chapters and to Linda Lien for typing, correcting, and duplicating countless versions of the manuscript. I also wish to thank Joan Catapano and the editorial staff at Indiana University Press for their faith in the project and their thoughtful efforts during each step of the publication process.

Portions of the following chapters originally appeared in a different form as articles in various journals:

Chapter 1: "Revisioning Clinical Research: Gender and the Ethics of Experimental Design," *Hypatia* 4, no. 2 (Summer 1989):125–139.

Chapter 2: "AIDS and Women," *AIDS Education and Prevention* 3, no. 3 (Fall 1991):230–240.

Chapter 3: "Is There Androcentric Bias in Psychiatric Diagnosis?" *The Journal of Medicine and Philosophy* 17 (1992):215–231.

Chapter 7: "Ignored, Overlooked, or Subsumed: Research on Lesbian Health and Health Care," *NWSA Journal* 5, no. 2 (Summer 1993):183–203. Appears here with permission from Ablex Publishing Corp.

Chapter 8: "Are There Feminist Methodologies Appropriate for the Natural Sciences and Do They Make a Difference?" *Women's Studies International Forum* 15, nos. 5/6 (1992):535–550. Appears here with kind permission from Pergamon Press Ltd, Headington Hill Hall, Oxford OX3 OBW, UK.

Chapter 9: "A Model for a Specialty in Women's Health," *Journal of Women's Health* 2, no. 2 (1993):99–104. It also appeared in a slightly modified version under the title "Women's Studies: A Model for a Specialty in Women's Health," *Transformations* 4, no. 1 (Spring 1993):9–18.

Introduction

Medicine and the health care system in the United States are currently facing a major crisis. Spiraling costs coupled with shortages of personnel, the rapid increase in chronic, incurable diseases, and the frustrations of patients have led to a call for national health care reform.

As a continuous stream of newspaper articles has revealed, women are the forgotten gender in much health research. Initial reports focused attention on basic research using male animal models, the theories and conclusions drawn from which might be problematic when extrapolated to female lower animals or human beings. More recent examinations suggest that clinical health research in humans suffers from some of the same flaws as basic research. The selection and definition of problems for study, the choice of experimental subjects, and conclusions drawn from the data in clinical trials often fail to include women or women's changing needs throughout the life span. For example, although heart disease is the biggest killer of both sexes, the 22,071 doctors included in the seven-year study of the effects of aspirin on cardiovascular disease were all men (Steering Committee of the Physician's Health Study Group, 1989). Little study has been undertaken on AIDS in women despite the fact that women constitute the group in which AIDS is currently increasing most rapidly. Women also appear to manifest different symptoms of AIDS. Since the progress of the disease has not been adequately studied and the Centers for Disease Control case definition failed until January 1993 to include gynecologic conditions related to AIDS in women, women tend to be diagnosed later than men (Rosser, 1991). The average life expectancy after diagnosis for a male is thirty months; for a woman it is fifteen weeks. The incidence of breast cancer, a deadly disease which occurs primarily in women, increased 24 percent between 1979 and 1986 (Grimes, 1991).

Mounting evidence reveals that access to health care also differs in accordance with gender as well as race, class, and age. Although a variety of factors contribute to this situation, it may be that bias in clinical research is reflected in bias in access to treatment. Women with kidney failure are less likely than men (30–50 percent depending upon the study) to receive an organ transplant. In one study only 4 percent of women with an abnormal report from a special heart scan were referred for a cardiac catheterization; 40 percent of men with an abnormal report were referred for the procedure (Steingart et al., 1991). Ten times as many women as men die in the hospital after angioplasty (Kelsey et al., 1993). Women who are poor, Black, and elderly often face insurmountable obstacles with the health care system even when they have been diagnosed with a known killer such as breast cancer.

The physician is placed in a difficult position. Because of the dearth of clinical research on those groups that now constitute the majority of the American population, s/he possesses inadequate information on the etiology, symptoms, and progress of many diseases in a population which is increasingly elderly, minority, and female. Emphasis upon synthesis of data analyzed by high-technology processes and instrumentation combined with the pressures to keep costs down by seeing patients quickly discourages physicians from talking and interacting extensively with patients.

Because the physician symbolizes medicine in the United States, s/he has become the target for the wrath of people wanting to vent their frustrations with the country's health care system. For example, the number of malpractice suits brought against physicians has increased dramatically. In addition, numerous polls, news articles, and headlines express the decreasing confidence of health care consumers in their physicians. For a *Newsweek* poll, the Gallup Organization interviewed 755 adults by telephone on March 25–26, 1993. Fifty percent of the people questioned stated that cost was their biggest concern about health care (37 percent stated quality and 11 percent availability). In response to the question, "How much blame should doctors bear for today's health care crisis?" 60 percent responded "most" or "some," while 35 percent thought other groups were mostly at fault (*Newsweek*, 1993, p. 28). Eighty-one percent agree that doctors in general charge too much, and 46 percent feel doctors make people wait too long for appointments, although they feel somewhat more positive about their own physician (*Newsweek*, 1993, p. 30).

Medical education must prepare students to deal with this crisis while continuing to produce competent, reliable physicians. Solutions for many of the problems are beyond the immediate reach of medical schools and the direct impact of medical education. Resources to deal with the increasing costs of health care must be found by insurance companies, employers, and other groups within the corporate and government sectors as suggested by government policies for health care reform.

Fortunately, solutions for other aspects of the crisis can be found within the pool of students currently receiving their medical education, in the persons of the women and people of color being trained to become physicians. During the past two decades the demographics of the group of medical students has changed drastically. In 1992–93, 41.6 percent of first-year medical students were women, compared to 9.2 percent in 1969–70 (Bickel and Quinnie, 1992). Although women in 1990 constitute only 17 percent of all practicing physicians (Bickel and Quinnie, 1992) and remain concentrated in the specialties of internal and general medicine, pediatrics, and psychiatry, the large number of women in medical school, coupled with the increasing numbers of women in residencies in all specialties, signals a dramatic change in the composition of practicing physicians.

As more women have entered medicine, medical schools and clinical hospitals have been forced to rethink traditional approaches and procedures such as the possibility of more flexible schedules. Although initiated for women, these changes frequently lead to superior education and clinical training for both male and female students and residents.

Similarly, as more women physicians have begun to practice medicine and reach theoretical and decision-making positions within the profession, positive effects from their perspective are beginning to be felt. Women have critiqued the male-centered focus of clinical research that has led to the insufficient study and funding of diseases of women, the exclusion of women from experimental drug trials, and the failure to understand the health of the elderly, who are mostly female.

This volume explores both the critiques resulting from male-focused medical research and health care practice and the solutions available to medical education which move women in to share the central focus. Following an introductory general critique of the ethical problems raised by an androcentric focus in clinical research, subsequent chapters in Part I examine the problems such a focus raises in internal medicine, psychiatry, and obstetrics and gynecology. The origins of the gender bias in clinical specialty research are traced to their roots in the related basic science discipline. The three chapters of Part II underline the particularly dramatic effects that the neglect of women's health in general has for particular subpopulations of women. Virtually no research has acknowledged the diversity among women; minority women, lesbians, and elderly women have largely been ignored in the scant research that has centered on women's health needs. In Part III, solutions are proposed through explorations of changes in methodologies, curriculum, classroom and clinical climate, teaching methods, and evaluation in medical education.

Emphasizing women in medical education would not only improve the situation for women physicians and patients, it would improve the situation for all. Male physicians need an inclusive education to create better professional relationships with their female colleagues and to gain the knowledge they need to treat the majority of the American population which is female and will continue to be increasingly elderly and minority. Women deserve to share central focus in the health care system. Since women are the bearers of both male and female children, the health of the nation depends on the health of its women.

REFERENCES

American Medical Association. 1990. *Physician characteristics and distribution in the U.S.* Chicago: American Medical Association.

Bickel, Janet, and Quinnie, Renee. 1992. *Women in medicine statistics.* Washington, D.C.: Association of American Medical Colleges.

Grimes, Charlotte. 1991. Health research often overlooks female gender. *St. Louis Post Dispatch,* April 28.

Kelsey, Sheryl F., et al., and Investigators from the National Heart, Lung, and Blood Institute Percutaneous Transluminal Coronary Angioplasty Registry.

1993. Results of percutaneous transluminal coronary angioplasty in women: 1985–1986 National Heart, Lung, and Blood Institutes Coronary Angioplasty Registry. *Circulation* 87, no. 3:720–727.

Newsweek poll. 1993. Doctors under the knife. *Newsweek,* April 5, pp. 28–33.

Rosser, Sue V. 1991. "AIDS and women." *AIDS Education and Prevention* 3, no. 3:230–240.

Steering Committee of the Physician's Health Study Group. 1989. Final report on the aspirin component of the ongoing physician's health study. *New England Journal of Medicine* 321:129–135.

Steingart, R. M.; Packer, M.; Hamm, P.; et al. 1991. Sex differences in the management of coronary artery disease. *New England Journal of Medicine* 325:226–230.

Part One

CRITIQUES OF THE ANDROCENTRIC FOCUS IN CLINICAL RESEARCH AND PRACTICE

CHAPTER ONE

Androcentric Bias in Clinical Research

In scientific research, whether it be in the behavioral, biomedical, or physical sciences, researchers rarely admit that data have been gathered and interpreted from a particular perspective. Since research in biology, chemistry, and physics centers on the physical and natural world, it is presumed to be "objective"; therefore, the term "perspective" does not apply to it. The reliability and repeatability of data gathered and hypotheses tested using the scientific method convince researchers that they are obtaining unbiased information about the physical, natural world.

Most researchers in the behavioral, biomedical, and physical sciences are trained in the scientific method and believe in its power. Few, however, are aware of its historical and philosophical roots in logical positivism and objectivity. Positivism implies that "all knowledge is constructed by inference from immediate sensory experiences" (Jaggar, 1983, pp. 355–356). It is premised on the assumption that human beings are highly individualistic and obtain knowledge in a rational manner that may be separated from their social conditions. This leads to the belief in the possibilities of obtaining knowledge that is both objective and value-free, the cornerstone of the scientific method.

Scientists, like all scholars, hold, either explicitly or implicitly, certain beliefs about their enterprise. Most believe, for example, that the laws and facts gathered by scientists are constant, providing that experiments have been done correctly. Historians of science posit that, quite to the contrary, the individuals who make observations and create theories are people who live in a particular country during a certain time in a definable socioeconomic condition, and thus their situations and mentalities inevitably impinge on their discoveries. Even their "facts" are contingent. Aristotle "counted" fewer teeth in the mouths of women than in those of men—adding this dentitional inferiority to all the others (Arditti, 1980). Galen, having read the book of Genesis, "discovered" that men had one less rib on one side than women did (Webster and Webster, 1974). Clearly, observation of what would appear by today's standards to be easily verifiable facts can vary depending upon the theory or paradigm by which the scientist is influenced.

Although every scientist strives to remain as neutral and value-free as possible, most scientists, feminists, and philosophers of science recognize that no individual can be completely objective. Instead "objectivity is defined to mean independence from the value judgments of any particular individual" (Jaggar, 1983, p. 357). The paradigms themselves, however, also are far from value-free. The present values of the culture and its history heavily influence the ordering of observable phenomena into theory. The world view of a particular society, time, and person limits the questions that can be asked and thereby the answers that can be given. Kuhn (1970) has demonstrated that the very acceptance of a particular paradigm that may appear to cause a "scientific revolution" within a society depends in fact upon the congruence of that theory with the institutions and beliefs of the society.

Longino (1990) has explored the extent to which methods employed by scientists can be objective and lead to repeatable, verifiable results while contributing to hypotheses or theories that are congruent with nonobjective institutions and ideologies of the society. "Background assumptions are the means by which contextual values and ideology are incorporated into scientific inquiry" (1990, p. 216). The institutions and beliefs of our society reflect the fact that the society is patriarchal. Even female scientists have only recently become aware of the influence of patriarchal bias in the paradigms of science.

In the past two decades, feminist historians and philosophers of science (Fee, 1981, 1982; Harding, 1986; Haraway, 1978, 1989; Longino, 1990) and feminist scientists (Bleier, 1984, 1986; Fausto-Sterling, 1985; Birke, 1986; Keller, 1983, 1985; and Rosser, 1988) have pointed out the bias and absence of value neutrality in science, particularly biology. By excluding females as experimental subjects, focusing on problems of primary interest to males, utilizing faulty experimental designs, and interpreting data based in language or ideas constricted by patriarchal parameters, scientists have introduced bias or flaws into their experimental results in several areas of biology. These flaws and biases were permitted to become part of the mainstream of scientific thought and were perpetuated in the scientific literature for decades. Because most scientists were men, values held by them as males were not distinguished as biasing; rather they were congruent with the values of all scientists and thus became synonymous with the "objective" view of the world (Keller, 1982, 1985).

A first step for feminist scientists was recognizing the possibility that androcentric bias would result from having virtually all theoretical and decision-making positions in science held by men (Keller, 1982). Not until a substantial number of women had entered the profession (Rosser, 1986) could this androcentrism be exposed. As long as only a few women were scientists, they had to demonstrate or conform to the male view of the world in order to be successful and have their research meet the criteria for "objectivity."

Once the possibility of androcentric bias was discovered, feminist scientists set out to explore the extent to which it had distorted science. They recognized potential distortion on a variety of levels of research and theory: the choice and definition of problems to be studied, the exclusion of females as experimental subjects, bias in the methodology used to collect and interpret data, and bias in theories and conclusions drawn from the data. They also began to realize that since the practice of modern medicine depends heavily on clinical research, any flaws and ethical problems in this research are likely to result in poorer health care and inequity in the medical treatment of disadvantaged groups. Recent evidence suggests that gender bias may have flawed some medical research.

CHOICE AND DEFINITION OF PROBLEMS FOR STUDY

With the expense of sophisticated equipment, maintenance of laboratory animals and facilities, and salaries for qualified technicians and researchers, virtually no medical research is undertaken today without federal or foundation support. Gone are the days when individuals had laboratories in their homes or made significant discoveries working in isolation using home-made equipment. In fiscal year 1989, the National Institutes of Health (NIH) funded approximately $7.1 billion in research (*Science and Government Report,* 1990). Private foundations and state governments funded a smaller portion (*National Science Foundation,* 1987).

The choice of problems for study in medical research is substantially determined by a national agenda that defines what is worthy of study, i.e., funding. As Marxist (Zimmerman et al., 1980), African-American (McLeod, 1987), and feminist (Hubbard, 1990) critics of scientific research have pointed out, the research that is undertaken reflects the societal bias toward the powerful, who are overwhelmingly white, middle- to upper-class, and male in the United States. Obviously, the majority of the members of Congress, who appropriate the funds for NIH and other federal agencies, fit this description; they are more likely to vote funds for health research which they view as beneficial as defined from their perspective.

It may be argued that actual priorities for medical research and allocations of funds are set not by members of Congress but by the leaders in medical research who are employees of NIH or other federal agencies or who are brought in as consultants. Unfortunately the same descriptors—white, middle- to upper-class, and male—tend to characterize the individuals in the theoretical and decision-making positions within the medical hierarchy and scientific establishment.

Having a preponderance of male leaders setting the priorities for medical research results in definite effects on the choice and definition of problems for research: Hypotheses are not formulated to focus on gender as a crucial part of the question being asked. Because it is clear that many diseases have different frequencies (heart disease, lupus), symptoms (gonorrhea), or complications (most sexually transmitted diseases) in the two sexes, scientists should routinely consider and test for differences or lack thereof based on gender in any hypothesis being tested. For example, when exploring the metabolism of a particular drug, tests should routinely be run in both males and females.

Five dramatic, widely publicized recent examples demonstrate that sex differences are *not* routinely considered as part of the question asked. In a longitudinal study of the effects of a cholesterol-lowering drug, gender differences were not tested; the drug was tested on 3,806 men and no women (Hamilton, 1985). The Multiple Risk Factor Intervention Trial (1990) examined mortality from coronary heart disease in 12,866 men only. The Health Professionals Follow-Up Study (Grobbee et al., 1990) looked at the association between coffee consumption and heart disease in 45,589 men. The Physician's Health Study (Steering Committee of the Physician's Health Study Group, 1989) found that low-dose aspirin therapy reduced the risk of myocardial infarction in 22,071 men. A study published in September 1992 in the *Journal of the American Medical Association* surveyed the literature from 1960 to 1991 on studies of clinical trials of medications used to treat acute myocardial infarction. Women were included in only about 20 percent of those studies; elderly people (over seventy-five years) were included in only 40 percent (Gurwitz, Nananda, and Avorn, 1992).

Some diseases which affect both sexes are defined as male diseases. Heart disease has been so designated because at younger ages it occurs more frequently in men than in women. Therefore, most of the funding for heart disease has been appropriated for research on predisposing factors (such as cholesterol level, lack of exercise, stress, smoking, and weight) using white, middle-aged, middle-class males.

This "male disease" designation has resulted in very little research being directed toward high-risk groups of women. Heart disease is a leading cause of death in older women (Kirschstein, 1985; Healy, 1991), who live an average of eight years longer than men (Boston Women's Health Book Collective, 1984). It is also frequent in poor African-American women who have had several children (Manley et al., 1985). Virtually no research has explored predisposing factors for these groups who fall outside the disease definition established from an androcentric perspective.

Recent data indicate that the designation of AIDS as a disease of male homosexuals and IV drug users has led to a failure among researchers and health care practitioners to understand the etiology and diagnosis of AIDS in women (Norwood, 1988). AIDS is currently increasing more rapidly among women than in any other group, and women appear to manifest different symptoms of AIDS than men. However, it was not until October 1992 that the Centers for Disease Control (CDC) announced a case definition that includes gynecologic conditions and other symptoms of AIDS in women; this case definition was enacted in January 1993 (Bell, 1993).

Research on conditions specific to females is accorded low priority, funding, and prestige, despite the fact that women make up half of the population and receive more than half of the health care. In 1988, the NIH allocated only 13.5 percent of its total budget to research on illnesses of major consequence to women (Narrigan, 1991). The Women's Health Initiative, launched by NIH in 1991 to study cardiovascular diseases, cancers, and osteoporosis, is attempting to raise the priority of women's health and provide baseline data on previously understudied causes of death in women (Pinn and LaRosa, 1992). Additional examples that might be targeted include dysmenorrhea, incontinence in older women, nutrition in postmenopausal women, and effects of exercise level and duration upon alleviation of menstrual discomfort. The issue of exposure to VDTs, which has resulted in "clusters" of women in certain industries giving birth to deformed babies, has also received low priority. In contrast, significant amounts of time and money are expended upon clinical research on women's bodies in connection with other aspects of reproduction. In this century up until the 1970s, considerable attention was devoted to the development of contraceptive devices for females rather than for males (Cowan, 1980; Dreifus, 1978). Furthermore, substantial clinical research has resulted in increasing medicalization and control of pregnancy, labor, and childbirth. Feminists have critiqued (Ehrenreich and English, 1978; Holmes, 1981) the conversion of a normal, natural process controlled by women into a clinical, and often surgical, procedure controlled by men. More recently, the new reproductive technologies such as amniocentesis, in vitro fertilization, and artificial insemination have become a major focus as means are sought to overcome infertility. Feminists (Arditti, Duelli Klein, and Minden, 1984; Corea and Ince, 1987; Corea et al., 1987; Klein, 1989) have warned of the extent to which these technologies place pressure on women to produce a "perfect" child while placing control in the hands of the male medical establishment.

These examples suggest that considerable resources and attention are devoted to women's health issues when those issues are directly related to men's interest in controlling the production of children. Contraceptive research may permit men to have sexual pleasure without the worry of producing children. Research on infertility, pregnancy, and childbirth has allowed men to assert more control over the production of more "perfect" children and over an aspect of women's lives over which they previously held less power.

Suggestions of fruitful questions for research based on the personal experience of women have also been ignored. In the health care area, women have often reported (and accepted among themselves) experiences that could not be documented by scientific experiments or were not accepted as valid by the researchers of the day. For decades, dysmenorrhea was attributed by most health care researchers and practitioners to psychological or social factors despite reports from an overwhelming number of women that these were monthly experiences in their lives. Only after prostaglandins were "discovered" was there widespread acceptance among the male medical establishment that this experience reported by women had a biological component (Kirschstein, 1985).

These four types of bias raise ethical issues. Health care practitioners must treat the majority of the population, which is female, based on information gathered from clinical research in which drugs may not have been tested on females, in which the etiology of the disease in women has not been studied, and in which women's experience has been ignored.

APPROACHES AND METHODS

The scientific community has often failed to include females in animal studies in both basic and clinical research unless the research centered on controlling the production of children. While the reasons for this exclusion (cleaner data from males due to lack of interference from estrous or menstrual cycles, fear of inducing fetal deformities in pregnant subjects, and higher incidence of some diseases in males) may be viewed as practical from a financial standpoint, it results in drugs that have not been adequately tested in women subjects before being marketed and a lack of information about the etiology of some diseases in women.

Using males as experimental subjects not only ignores the fact that females may respond differently to the variable tested, it may also lead to less accurate models even in the male. Models which more accurately simulate functioning of complex biological systems may be derived by using female rats or primates as subjects in experiments. With the exception of insulin and the hormones of the female reproductive cycle, traditional endocrinological theory assumed that most of the twenty-odd human hormones are maintained at a constant level in both males and females. Thus, the male of the species was chosen as the experimental subject because of his noncyclicity. However, new techniques of measuring blood hormone levels have demonstrated episodic, rather than steady, patterns of secretion of virtually all hormones in both males and females. As Joan Hoffman (1982) points out, the rhythmic cycle of hormone secretion as also portrayed in the cycling female rat appears to be a more accurate model for the secretion of most hormones.

When females have been used as experimental subjects, often they have been treated as not fully human. In his attempts to investigate the side effects (Goldzieher et al., 1971a) of nervousness and depression (Goldzieher et al., 1971b) attributable to oral contraceptives, Goldzieher gave dummy pills to seventy-six women who sought treatment at a San Antonio clinic to prevent further pregnancies. None of the women was told that she was participating in research or receiving placebos (Veatch, 1971; Cowan, 1980). The women in Goldzieher's study were primarily poor, multiparous Mexican-Americans. Research that raises similar questions about the ethics of informed consent was carried out on poor Puerto Rican women during the initial phases of testing the effectiveness of the birth control pill as a contraceptive (Zimmerman et al., 1980). Recent data have revealed routine testing of pregnant women for HIV positivity without their informed consent at certain clinics (Marte and Anastos, 1990; Chavkin, Driver, and Forman, 1989) and subsequent pressure placed on women who are HIV-positive to abort their fetuses (Selwyn et al., 1989).

Frequently it is difficult to determine whether these women are treated as less than human because of their gender or whether race and class are more significant variables. The Tuskegee Syphilis Experiment, in which the effects of untreated syphilis were studied in 399 men over a period of forty years (Jones, 1981), made it clear that poor African-American men may not receive appropriate treatment or information about the experiment in which they are participating. Feminist scholars (Dill, 1983; Ruzek, 1988) have begun to explore the extent to which gender, race, and class may become complex, interlocking political variables affecting access to and quality of health care.

Current clinical research sets up a distance between the observer and the human subject being studied. Several feminist philosophers (Keller, 1985; Hein, 1981; Haraway, 1978; Harding, 1986) have characterized this as an androcentric approach. Distance between the observer and experimental subject may be more comfortable for men, who are raised to feel more at ease with autonomy and distance (Keller, 1985), than for women, who tend to value relationships and interdependency (Gilligan, 1982).

Using only the methods traditional to a particular discipline may result in limited approaches that fail to reveal sufficient information about the problem being explored. This may be a particular difficulty for research surrounding medical problems of pregnancy, childbirth, menstruation, and menopause, for which the methods of one discipline are clearly inadequate.

Methods which cross disciplinary boundaries or include combinations of methods traditionally used in separate fields may be more appropriate. For example, if the topic of research is occupational exposures that present a risk to the pregnant woman working in a plant where toxic chemicals are manufactured, a combination of methods traditionally used in social science research with methods frequently used in biology and chemistry may be the best approach. Checking the chromosomes of any miscarried fetuses, chemical analysis of placentae after birth, Apgar scores of the babies at birth, and blood samples of the newborns to determine trace amounts of the toxic chemicals would be appropriate biological and chemical means of gathering data about the problem. In-depth interviews with women to discuss how they are feeling and any irregularities they detect during each month of the pregnancy, or weekly evaluation using written questionnaires regarding the pregnancy progress are methods more traditionally used in the social sciences for problems of this sort. Jean Hamilton has called for interactive models that draw on both the social and natural sciences to explain complex problems:

> Particularly for understanding human, gender-related health, we need more interactive and contextual models that address the actual complexity of the phenomenon that is the subject of explanation. One example is the need for more phenomenological definitions of symptoms, along with increased recognition that psychology, behavioral studies, and sociology are among the "basic sciences" for health research. Research on heart disease is one example of a field where it is recognized that both psychological stress and behaviors such as eating and cigarette smoking influence the onset and natural course of a disease process. (1985, VI-62)

Perhaps an increase in the number of women holding decision-making positions in the design and funding of clinical research would result in more interdisciplinary research on issues of women's health care such as menstruation, pregnancy, childbirth, lactation, and menopause. Those complex phenomena fall outside the range of methods of study provided by a sole discipline. Interdisciplinary approaches developed to solve these problems might then be applied to other complex problems to benefit all health care consumers, both male and female.

THEORIES AND CONCLUSIONS DRAWN FROM THE RESEARCH

The rationale which is traditionally presented in support of "objective" methods is that they prevent bias. Emphasis upon traditional disciplinary approaches that are quantitative and maintain the distance between observer and experimental subject supposedly eliminate bias on the part of the researcher. Ironically, to the extent that these "objective" approaches are synonymous with a masculine approach to the world, they may actually introduce bias. Specifically, androcentric bias may permeate the theories and conclusions drawn from the research in several ways:

Theories may be presented in androcentric language. Much feminist scholarship has focused on problems of sexism in language and the extent to which patriarchal language has excluded and limited women (Thorne, 1979; Lakoff, 1975; Kramarae and Treichler, 1986). Sexist language is a symptom of underlying sexism, but language also shapes our concepts and provides the framework through which we express our ideas. Being aware of sexism and the limitations of patriarchal language may allow feminist researchers to describe their observations in less gender-biased terms.

The limited research on AIDS in women has focused on women as prostitutes or mothers. Describing the woman as a vector for transmission to men (prostitute) or the fetus (mother) has produced little information on the progress of AIDS in women themselves (Rosser, 1991). Once the bias in the terminology is exposed, the next step is to ask whether that terminology leads to a constraint or bias in the theory itself.

An androcentric perspective may lead to the formulation of theories and conclusions drawn from medical research to support the status quo of inequality for women and other oppressed groups. Building upon their awareness of these biases, women scientists have critiqued studies of brain-hormone interaction (Bleier, 1984) for their biological determinism used to justify women's socially inferior position. Bleier repeatedly warned against extrapolating from one species to another in biochemical as well as behavioral traits (Bleier, 1986).

Not surprisingly, the androcentric bias in research which has led to the exclusion of women from the definitions of and approaches to research problems has resulted in differences in the management of disease and access to health care procedures based on gender. In a 1991 study in Massachusetts and Maryland, Ayanian and Epstein (1991) demonstrated that women were significantly less likely than men to undergo coronary angioplasty, angiography, or surgery when admitted to the hospital with the diagnosis of myocardial infarction, unstable angina, chronic ischemic heart disease, or chest pain. This significant difference remained even when variables such as race, age, economic status, and other chronic diseases such as diabetes and heart failure were controlled for. A similar study (Steingart et al., 1991) revealed that women had angina before myocardial infarction as frequently as and with more debilitating effects than men, yet women are referred for cardiac catheterization only half as often. The 1992 *Journal of the American Medical Association* study concluded that the exclusion of women from 80 percent of the trials and of the elderly from 60 percent of the trials for medication for myocardial infarction limits the ability to generalize study findings to the patient population that experiences the most morbidity and mortality from acute myocardial infarction (Gurwitz, Nananda, and Avorn, 1992). Gender bias in cardiac research has therefore been translated into bias in the management of disease, leading to inequitable treatment for life-threatening conditions in women.

Androcentric bias in AIDS research may also lead to underdiagnosis and higher death rates for women. Because the progress of AIDS in women has not been adequately studied, and since the CDC case definition for AIDS failed until very recently to include any gynecologic conditions, most health care workers are unable to diagnose AIDS in women until the disease has advanced significantly. On average, men die thirty months after diagnosis, women fifteen weeks. Theories and conclusions drawn from AIDS research should be examined to determine to what extent they represent and reinforce sexism, racism, and classism.

Recognizing the possibility of gender bias is the first step toward understanding the difference it makes. Perhaps male researchers are less likely to see flaws in and question biologically deterministic theories that provide scientific justification for men's superior status in society because they gain social power and status from such theories. Researchers from outside the mainstream (women, for example) are much more likely to be critical of such theories because they lose power from them. To eliminate bias, the community of scientists undertaking clinical research needs to include individuals from backgrounds as varied and diverse as possible with regard to race, class, gender, and sexual orientation (Rosser, 1988). Only then is it less likely that the perspective of one group will bias research design, approaches, subjects, and interpretations.

However, given that the overall agenda for research policies concerning access to health care is set in the political arena, politicians must also reflect the diversity and needs of the population. Then we can work together to overcome gender bias in health research.

REFERENCES

Arditti, Rita. 1980. Feminism and science. In Rita Arditti, Pat Brennan, and Steve Cavrak (eds.), *Science and liberation.* Boston: South End Press.

Arditti, Rita; Duelli Klein, Renate; and Minden, Shelley. 1984. *Test-tube women: What future for motherhood?* London: Pandora Press.

Ayanian, J. Z., and Epstein, A. M. 1991. Differences in the use of procedures between women and men hospitalized for coronary heart disease. *New England Journal of Medicine* 325:221–225.

Bell, Nora. 1993. Board of the National Leadership Coalition on AIDS. Personal communication.

Birke, Lynda. 1986. *Women, feminism, and biology.* New York: Methuen.

Bleier, Ruth. 1984. *Science and gender: A critique of biology and its theories on women.* New York: Pergamon Press.

———. 1986. Sex differences research: Science or belief? In Ruth Bleier (ed.), *Feminist approaches to science.* New York: Pergamon Press.

Boston Women's Health Book Collective. 1984. *The new our bodies, ourselves.* New York: Simon and Schuster.

Chavkin, W.; Driver, C.; and Forman, P. 1989. The crisis in New York City's perinatal services. *New York State Journal of Medicine* 89, no. 12:658–663.

Corea, G., et al. (eds.). 1987. *Man-made women: How new reproductive technologies affect women.* Bloomington: Indiana University Press.

Corea, Gena, and Ince, S. 1987. Report of a survey of IVF clinics in the U.S. In Patricia Spallone and Deborah L. Steinberg (eds.), *Made to order: The myth of reproductive and genetic progress.* Oxford: Pergamon Press.

Cowan, Belita. 1980. Ethical problems in government-funded contraceptive research. In Helen Holmes, Betty Hoskins, and Michael Gross (eds.), *Birth control and controlling birth: Women-centered perspectives,* pp. 37–46. Clifton, N.J.: Humana Press.

Dill, Bonnie T. 1983. Race, class and gender: Prospects for an all-inclusive sisterhood. *Feminist Studies* 9:1.

Dreifus, Claudia. 1978. *Seizing our bodies.* New York: Vintage Books.

Ehrenreich, Barbara, and English, Deirdre. 1978. *For her own good.* New York: Anchor Press.

Fausto-Sterling, Anne. 1985. *Myths of gender.* New York: Basic Books.

Fee, Elizabeth. 1981. Is feminism a threat to scientific objectivity? *International Journal of Women's Studies* 4:213–233.

———. 1982. A feminist critique of scientific objectivity. *Science for the People* 14, no. 4:8.

Gilligan, Carol. 1982. *In a different voice: Psychological theory and women's development.* Cambridge, Mass.: Harvard University Press.

Goldzieher, Joseph W.; Moses, Louis; Averkin, Eugene; Scheel, Cora; and Taber, Ben. 1971a. A placebo-controlled double-blind crossover investigation of the side effects attributed to oral contraceptives. *Fertility and Sterility* 22, no. 9:609–623.

———. 1971b. Nervousness and depression attributed to oral contraceptives: A double-blind, placebo-controlled study. *American Journal of Obstetrics and Gynecology* 22:1013–1020.

Grobbee, D. E., et al. 1990. Coffee, caffeine, and cardiovascular disease in men. *New England Journal of Medicine* 321:1026–1032.

Gurwitz, Jerry H.; Nananda, F. Colonel; and Avorn, Jerry. 1992. The exclusion of the elderly and women from clinical trials in acute myocardial infarction. *Journal of the American Medical Association* 268, no. 2:1417–1422.

Hamilton, Jean. 1985. Avoiding methodological biases in gender-related research. In *Women's health report of the Public Health Service Task Force on Women's Health Issues.* Washington, D.C.: U.S. Department of Health and Human Service Public Service.

Haraway, Donna. 1978. Animal sociology and a natural economy of the body politic, Part I: A political physiology of dominance; and Animal sociology and a natural economy of the body politic, Part II: The past is the contested zone: Human nature and theories of production and reproduction in primate behavior studies. *Signs: Journal of Women in Culture and Society* 4, no. 1:21–60.

———. 1989. Monkeys, aliens, and women: Love, science, and politics at the intersection of feminist theory and colonial discourse. *Women's Studies International Forum* 12, no. 3:295–312.

Harding, Sandra. 1986. *The science question in feminism.* Ithaca, N.Y.: Cornell University Press.

Healy, Bernadine. 1991. Women's health, public welfare. *Journal of the American Medical Association* 264, no. 4:566–568.

Hein, Hilde. 1981. Women and science: Fitting men to think about nature. *International Journal of Women's Studies* 4:369–377.

Hoffman, J. C. 1982. Biorhythms in human reproduction: The not-so-steady states. *Signs: Journal of Women in Culture and Society* 7, no. 4:829–844.

Holmes, Helen B. 1981. Reproductive technologies: The birth of a women-centered analysis. In Helen B. Holmes et al. (eds.), *The custom-made child?* Clifton, N.J.: Humana Press.

Hubbard, Ruth. 1990. *The politics of women's biology.* New Brunswick, N.J.: Rutgers University Press.

Jaggar, Alison M. 1983. *Feminist politics and human nature.* Totowa, N.Y.: Rowman and Allanheld.

Jones, James H. 1981. *Bad blood: The Tuskegee syphilis experiment.* New York: The Free Press.

Keller, Evelyn Fox. 1982. Feminism and science. *Signs: Journal of Women in Culture and Society* 7, no. 3:589–602.

———. 1983. *A feeling for the organism: The life and work of Barbara McClintock.* New York: W. H. Freeman.

———. 1985. *Reflections on gender and science.* New Haven, Conn.: Yale University Press.

Kirschstein, Ruth L. 1985. *Women's health: Report of the Public Health Service Task Force on Women's Health Issues.* Vol. 2. Washington, D.C.: U.S. Department of Health and Human Services Public Health Service.

Klein, Renate D. 1989. *Infertility.* London: Pandora Press.

Kramarae, Cheris, and Treichler, Paula. 1986. *A feminist dictionary.* London: Pandora Press.

Kuhn, Thomas S. 1970. *The structure of scientific revolutions.* 2nd ed. Chicago: The University of Chicago Press.

Lakoff, Robin. 1975. *Language and woman's place.* New York: Harper and Row Publishers, Inc.

Longino, Helen. 1990. *Science as social knowledge: Values and objectivity in scientific inquiry.* Princeton, N.J.: Princeton University Press.

Manley, Audrey; Lin-Fu, Jane; Miranda, Magdalena; Noonan, Alan; and Parker, Tanya. 1985. Special health concerns of ethnic minority women in women's health. *Report of the Public Health Service Task Force on Women's Health Issues.* Washington, D.C.: U.S. Department of Health and Human Services.

Marte, C., and Anastos, K. 1990. Women—the missing persons in the AIDS epidemic. Part II. *Health/PAC Bulletin* 20, no. 1:11–23.

McLeod, S. 1987. *Scientific colonialism: A cross-cultural comparison.* Washington, D.C.: Smithsonian Institution Press.

Money, John, and Erhardt, Anke. 1972. *Man and woman, boy and girl.* Baltimore: Johns Hopkins University Press.

Multiple Risk Factor Intervention Trial Research Group. 1990. Mortality rates after 10.5 years for participants in the Multiple Risk Factor Intervention Trial: Findings related to a prior hypothesis of the trial. *Journal of the American Medical Association* 263:1795–1801.

Narrigan, Deborah. 1991. Research to improve women's health: An agenda for equity. *The Network News: National Women's Health Network* (March/April/May):3, 9.

National Science Foundation. 1987. *Science and Engineering Indicators.* NSB-1, Appendix Table 4–10. Washington, D.C.: NSF.

Norwood, Chris. 1988. Alarming rise in deaths. *Ms.* (July):65–67.

Pinn, Vivian, and LaRosa, Judith. 1992. Overview: Office of research on women's health. *National Institutes of Health,* pp. 1–10.

Rosser, Sue V. 1986. *Teaching science and health from a feminist perspective: A practical guide.* Elmsford, N.Y.: Pergamon Press.

———. 1988. Women in science and health care: A gender at risk. In Sue V. Rosser (ed.), *Feminism within the science of health care professions: Overcoming resistance.* Elmsford, N.Y.: Pergamon Press.

———. 1991. AIDS and women. *AIDS Education and Prevention* 3, no. 3:230–240.

Ruzek, Sheryl. 1988. Women's health: Sisterhood is powerful, but so are race and class. Keynote addresss delivered at Southeast Women's Studies Association Annual Conference, February 27, University of North Carolina–Chapel Hill.

Science and government report. 1990. Washington, D.C., March 1, 18, no. 4:1.

Selwyn, P. A., et al. 1989. Prospective study of human immunodeficiency virus infection and pregnancy outcomes in intravenous drug users. *Journal of the American Medical Association* 261:1289–1294.

Steering Committee of the Physician's Health Study Research Group. 1988. Special report: Preliminary report of findings from the aspirin component of the ongoing physician's health study. *New England Journal of Medicine* 318, no. 4:262–264.

Steering Committee of the Physician's Health Study Group. 1989. Final report on the aspirin component of the ongoing physician's health study. *New England Journal of Medicine* 321:129–135.

Steingart, R. M.; Packes, M.; Hamm, P.; et al. 1991. Sex differences in the management of coronary artery disease. *New England Journal of Medicine* 325:226–230.

Thorne, Barrie. 1979. Claiming verbal space: Women, speech and language in college classrooms. Paper presented at the Research Conference on Educational Environments and the Undergraduate Women, September 13–15, Wellesley College.

Veatch, Robert M. 1971. *Experimental pregnancy.* Hastings Center Report 1:2–3.

Webster, Douglas, and Webster, Molly. 1974. *Comparative vertebrate morphology.* New York: Academic Press.

Zimmerman, B., et al. 1980. People's science. In Rita Arditti, Pat Brennan, and Steve Cavrak (eds.), *Science and liberation,* pp. 299–319. Boston: South End Press.

CHAPTER TWO

Underdiagnosis and Inadequate Treatment

AIDS and Women

Basic science research undergirds all aspects of clinical research. Biases that distort the choice and definition of problems for study, methods, and theories and conclusions drawn from the data in the basic science disciplines may result in similar biases in the research in related clinical specialties. Clinical research in AIDS must be interdisciplinary and combine social and medical specialties ranging from epidemiology through neurology to infectious diseases. The basic science research in immunology, the foundation for much of the clinical research, is rooted in cellular and molecular biology.

POSSIBLE SOURCES OF ANDROCENTRIC BIAS IN BASIC SCIENCE RESEARCH

Feminist critiques of cellular and molecular biology have helped to reveal the points where androcentric bias has undermined the foundations of basic science research in those fields. The patriarchal language and values of scientists and society inform the problems chosen for study and the theoretical concepts of the subdisciplines that examine cellular and molecular processes occurring below the organismal level. Critiques conclude that faulty research design, overextension of data, and generally "bad" science may be more acceptable in some research if they provide scientific bases for the social status quo.

The themes of reductionism and control have also dominated the study of cellular structure, physiology, and molecular interactions. In the earlier part of the twentieth century, various species ranging from the simple (bacteria) to more complex (corn, drosophila, mice) were used to study complexities of the cell. Both interactive and organizer models were proposed to explain development and functioning.

During the latter half of the century, control mechanisms in simpler organisms began to dominate the research funded and accepted as theoretically valid. One obvious influence on the direction of the research was the phenomenal increase in technologically sophisticated equipment which made it possible to see increasingly smaller structures in simple organisms. Evelyn Fox Keller (1983) points out the profound impact of the large number of physicists who entered the field of molecular biology, particularly after World War II. Trained as physicists, they transferred some of the tenets of physics—the emphasis on simplicity, deductive reasoning, and the search for universal laws that control—to molecular biology. In short, as Ruth Hubbard suggests, the physicists sought the answer to the question, "What is life?" by reducing living organisms to increasingly smaller units of chemistry and physics.

> I emphasize this reductionism because Watson has written that, long before they knew each other, he and Crick acquired their keen interest in genes and DNA by reading Erwin Schrodinger's (1944) *What Is Life?* Written by one of the great physicists, this little book drew the attention of physicists to biology at the end of World War II, when many of them were becoming disillusioned with physics. After all, by 1945, the proud physics of relativity and quantum theory and of the principles of complementarity and uncertainty had generated the atomic bombs that destroyed Hiroshima and Nagasaki. Intellectually as well, physics was beginning to degenerate into queuing up in front of bigger and bigger machines so as to produce smaller and smaller particles. Many physicists had begun to look for more interesting problems and responded to Schrodinger's challenge of the gene as the new frontier. (Hubbard, 1990, p. 53)

Feminist scientists (Keller, 1983; Hubbard, 1990; Birke, 1986; Fausto-Sterling, 1985, 1992; Bleier, 1984) have strongly criticized the Watson-Crick model of DNA as the "master molecule," calling it an androcentric view of the cell. The masculine world view that surrounded the "discovery" of the double helix as the control mechanism in the cell is well documented in Watson's (1969) own account of the event. Sayre (1975) exposed Watson and Crick's exclusion and shameful treatment of Rosalind Franklin and their failure to acknowledge her substantial contribution to their work as one facet of their androcentrism. Feminist philosophers of science (Haraway, 1978) and feminist scientists (Keller, 1983; Hubbard, 1990) have demonstrated the androcentrism of reductionism and control inherent in the idea that life can be reduced to the DNA on the genes in the nucleus. (Not coincidentally, as these writers note, this gives the father equal status, since he contributes DNA in amounts equal to that contributed by the mother to the developing cell.) They also point out that the hierarchical nature of the "central dogma" of DNA—RNA—Protein parallels the hierarchical organizational charts of corporate structures (Keller, 1985) with unidirectional information flow from the top down.

The congruence of this hierarchical, reductionistic model, which centers unidirectional control for all life processes in the DNA in the nucleus of the cell, with other social institutions such as corporations, the Catholic church, and the patriarchal family led scientists to accept this model despite increasing contradictory evidence. Alternative models which emphasize interaction between the nucleus and cytoplasm and interrelationships and process (Nanney, 1957; Thomas, 1974) were proposed by scientists representing a minority view during the "central dogma" era. Individuals who worked with more complex organisms (McClintock, 1950) warned that the Watson-Crick model did not explain the functioning of these organisms. The views of these scientists were and continue to be largely rejected, misunderstood, or ignored. Partially as a result of the biography of Barbara McClintock written by Evelyn Fox Keller (1983), more interactive models contradicting DNA as the master molecule are slowly being accepted. McClintock also rejected the predominant hierarchical theory of genetic DNA as the "master molecule" that controls gene action; she focused instead on the interaction between the organism and its environment as the locus of control.

Despite some growing recognition of the oversimplicity of the "master molecule" model of DNA and its failure to explain data from complex organisms, it continues to dominate the direction of much research in molecular biology. Most recently Watson has received billions of dollars, a large percentage of the budget of the National Institutes of Health, plus additional funding from other foundations, for the Human Genome Project. The Human Genome Project is an attempt to sequence (find the chemical structure of in, terms of base pairs of DNA) all twenty-three pairs of human chromosomes. The premise is that defects in genes cause diseases and syndromes, and that knowing the exact location of each gene on the chromosome and its molecular structure (which can be discovered through gene sequencing) is the first step toward being able to correct the gene and therefore cure the disease or defect.

In a time of tight fiscal constraints, spending billions of federal dollars for the Human Genome Project is a questionable use of resources for many reasons. It is reductionistic and controlling in that it isolates the gene (not even the gene's interaction with the environment) as the focus for disease. This is problematic in that genetic defects are responsible for only a small percentage of diseases. Even for those diseases such as cancer and cardiovascular disease which have genetic components, it is the interaction of those genetic components with environmental factors that determines who gets the disease. Most diseases and deaths in our society, however, are not due to genetic defects. Poverty, malnutrition, lack of education about prevention, and lack of access to existing medical care such as vaccination and prenatal care are the major causes of disease and death. By focusing on sequencing DNA in the chromosomes, the Human Genome Project diverts money from known cures for disease. It suggests a biological basis for problems that have social and economic causes in our society.

ANDROCENTRIC BIAS IN CLINICAL RESEARCH ON AIDS

The research on Acquired Immune Deficiency Syndrome (AIDS) demonstrates similar problems which may result when clinical studies reflect androcentrism and a lack of consideration for the interaction of social and biological factors in causing disease. AIDS is a prime example of a disease in which androcentrism has placed women at a disadvantage in diagnosis, treatment, and care. A considerable literature has begun to evolve about women and AIDS, ranging from its general epidemiology (Guinan and Hardy, 1987; Willoughby, 1989), through its incidence in particular groups of women such as prostitutes (Rosenberg and Weiner, 1988), drug-dependent women (Mondanaro, 1987), and pregnant women (Selwyn et al., 1989; Hand et al., 1989), to articles about the psychosocial and legal needs of women with AIDS (Zuckerman and Gordon, 1988). Recent literature reveals the extent to which women are the missing persons and victims of the AIDS epidemic (Anastos and Marte, 1989; Marte and Anastos, 1990) and are also shouldering a major burden as caregivers to individuals with the disease (World Health Organization Global Programme on AIDS, 1990). At the 9th International AIDS Conference held in Berlin, Germany, in 1993, it was reported by the World Health Organization that at least 40 percent of the four million AIDS infections in the world have occurred among women, and that in many nations the total among women exceeds the rate of infection among men (GayNet News Service, 1993).

One reason that women have been ignored in the AIDS epidemic in the United States is the initial mistake that was made in defining the disease by groups of individuals. The original designation of AIDS as a gay male disease, with the subsequent inclusion of intravenous drug users and Haitian immigrants, led to a lack of funding and study of AIDS and its transmission (Shilts, 1987) and diagnosis in many populations, including women.

AIDS is the leading cause of death for women aged twenty to forty in major cities in sub-Saharan Africa, the Americas, and Western Europe (Gillespie, 1991, p. 20). Even though women have been shown to be at least as likely as men to become victims of the disease, little funding and study have been directed toward diagnosis, etiology, and treatment for women. Although initial group designation may be responsible for some of this neglect, other factors such as equity of distribution of limited resources and utility/usefulness of the infected have further complicated decisions. For example, a February 1993 report, "The Social Impact of AIDS," issued by the National Research Council suggested targeting limited AIDS resources toward a "total of 23 to 30 neighborhoods in cities including San Francisco, Los Angeles, Houston, Miami, Newark, Camden, NJ, and New York City" (Kolata, 1993, A-1). Because the epidemic is "settling into spacially and socially isolated groups and possibly becoming endemic in them," the council recommended putting the money where the problem is (Kolata, 1993, A-1).

However, the androcentrism which dominates clinical research and medical practice in general may be as responsible as initial group designation. Male-centered perspectives that lead to choices of problems for study that ignore symptoms of disease in women and exclude females in experimental approaches and as subjects will lead to the underdiagnosis and treatment of women for most diseases outside of obstetrics/gynecology, where they may be overdiagnosed and overtreated. AIDS in women serves as a particularly dramatic example of an androcentric bias that leads to poor health care for women.

CHOICE AND DEFINITION OF PROBLEMS FOR STUDY

The effect of the national agenda on the choice of problems for study in medical research is reflected clearly in AIDS research. That agenda is substantially influenced by gender, race, class, and heterosexual privilege.

Although AIDS affects both sexes, it has been labeled a male disease in the United States. The facts that the disease was first identified in the male homosexual/bisexual population and that male homosexuals/bisexuals still constitute the largest proportion of AIDS cases clearly have contributed to this ascription. IV drug use, which is the second-leading risk behavior for AIDS transmission, is also more frequent in men than in women in the United States.

These statistical and historical reasons explain why the case definition for surveillance of AIDS (Centers for Disease Control, 1987) was initially based on characteristics found in males, and why most funding was originally directed toward studying the disease in men. What cannot be explained is why the focus did not shift to include women when the evidence regarding heterosexual intercourse as the major mode for transmission of AIDS in Africa and the statistical fact that AIDS in the United States is increasing most rapidly among Black and Hispanic women became known (CDC, 1990). Not until January 1993 was the CDC case definition changed to encompass symptoms common in women. When the first statistics using the more inclusive definition surfaced, "the number of people with AIDS increased at a surprising rate during the first three months of the year, when more than 35,000 new cases were reported" (The State, 4/30/93, A-3).

The continued designation of AIDS as a male disease further exemplifies the androcentrism which led to the inadequate study and identification of heart disease in high-risk groups of women because heart disease was defined as a male disease (Kirschstein, 1985; Healy, 1991). At the 9th Annual International AIDS conference in 1993, the U.S. Surgeon General released an explicit report with a new focus on the danger the epidemic poses for women. "Dr. Antonio Novello released the report at the AIDS conference, saying it had been ready for two years but that the Bush administration had refused to release it because it was too graphic" (Gaynet News Service, 1993, p. 10).

Nor has gender been a crucial consideration in the hypotheses for characterization or study of AIDS. Since it is clear that many diseases have different frequencies, symptoms, or complications in the two sexes, scientists should routinely consider and test for differences or lack thereof based on gender in any hypothesis being tested.

Several indicators suggest that clinical researchers and practitioners routinely fail to ask how AIDS might differ in women. Higher rates of abnormal Pap smears and cervical cancer in HIV-infected women compared to uninfected women (Provenchar et al., 1988; Schrager et al., 1989), increased incidence of pelvic inflammatory disease that resists treatment (Hoegsberg et al., 1988), and severe vaginal yeast infections resistant to cure (Rhoads et al., 1987) had been documented in HIV-positive women well before January 1993. Yet until that year none of these conditions was included in the CDC's revised case definition for AIDS (1987). Ironically, candidiasis (yeast infection) of the esophagus, trachea, bronchi, or lungs was listed as an indicator disease diagnosed definitively without laboratory evidence regarding HIV infection or as an indicator disease diagnosed presumptively with laboratory evidence for HIV infection. Women with AIDS are much more likely to experience vaginal yeast infections before clinical manifestations in other sites. It is difficult to understand why this symptom was not included in the CDC case definition before 1993 unless one recognizes the androcentric focus which leads to such oversights.

Additional evidence suggests that researchers have failed to ask how gender may differentially affect diagnosis in women. Norwood (1988) compiled statistics demonstrating dramatic, unexplained increases in deaths of women from a variety of respiratory and infectious diseases (154 percent in New York City; 225 percent in Washington, D.C.) from 1981 to 1986 in geographic areas in which AIDS is frequent in men. In areas with a low percentage of AIDS cases (Idaho, for example), no concurrent increases in women's deaths from unexplained respiratory and infectious diseases have occurred. Did focus on the etiology of pneumocystis carinii pneumonia (PCP), which is a major cause of AIDS deaths in males, lead practitioners to misunderstand subtle differences in manifestation of PCP in women and/or to underdiagnose PCP as a minor respiratory ailment when it occurred in women? The first-quarter statistics of AIDS cases in 1993 revealed a 204 percent increase over the previous year. Most of the increase is attributed to the broadened definition, which includes more symptoms of AIDS in women, thus substantiating earlier suggestions of underdiagnosis in women (Livingston, 1993).

Research on AIDS conditions specific to females has received low priority, funding, and prestige. Anastos and Marte (1989) suggest that fundamental questions about the progression of the disease in women have not been explored: "Is cervical cancer more common in HIV-infected women? How does HIV infection affect pregnancy and childbirth? Do the different hormones in women and men affect the course of HIV infection? Do women fall prey to different opportunistic infections than men do? Do women respond differently to treatment regimens established for male patients? Do women suffer different side effects and toxicities from AIDS medications? Do women survive a shorter time after the diagnosis of AIDS has been made? Are the causes of death in women different than in men?" (Anastos and Marte, 1989; p. 7). Although data (CDC, 1990) indicate that in the United States heterosexual transmission has produced a faster rate of increase in AIDS among women than in any other group, most funding and study are still directed toward men. A 1991 issue of *Ms.* states that neither of the two institutes distributing the funds for U.S. AIDS research has funded a major project to address whether women with AIDS may experience different symptoms than men. "Dr. Daniel Hoth, AIDS division director for the National Institute of Allergy and Infectious Diseases (NIAID), a man who controls millions of research dollars, reluctantly concedes he has sponsored no studies about women's health. And the situation is the same at the National Cancer Institute; together, the two institutes get the bulk of U.S. AIDS research dollars, but neither has gotten around to asking what AIDS looks like in women" (Byron, 1991, p. 24). A 1993 report revealed that in nine U.S. cities, AIDS was the leading cause of death for women ages twenty-five to forty-four (National News Roundup, 1993, p. 12).

This androcentric perspective also explains why the meager funding and study of AIDS in women has been directed primarily at two groups— pregnant women and prostitutes. Feminists (Rosser, 1989; Corea et al., 1987; and Ehrenreich and English, 1978) have pointed out that considerable funding and clinical research may be focused on women's health issues when those issues are directly related to men's interest in controlling the production of children.

A considerable portion of the research and literature on HIV infection in women is based on studies of prostitutes (Cohen et al., 1988; CDC, 1988; CDC, 1987). Rather than an attempt to understand the manifestations and progression of the disease in women, the focus of these studies has been epidemiological and the heterosexual transmission of AIDS to men. Anastos and Marte (1989) emphasize that comparable discussion about heterosexual transmission to women whose male partners have had multiple sexual encounters has not been aired in the literature. Studies demonstrate that the source of AIDS infection for most prostitutes is intravenous drug use, rather than sexual contact (Anastos and Marte, 1989).

As with the research on prostitutes, few of the studies on AIDS in pregnant women have examined the disease in the women except as it affects transmission to the fetus (Minkoff, Moreno, and Powderly, 1992). Recent data have revealed routine testing of pregnant women for HIV positivity without their informed consent at certain clinics (Marte and Anastos, 1990; Chavkin, Driver, and Forman, 1989), and subsequent pressure placed on women who are HIV-positive to abort their fetuses (Selwyn et al., 1989). Little attention is paid to the progress of the disease in the women themselves or to their suffering; instead the focus is on the product of conception.

The androcentric perspective biasing the choice and definition of problems chosen for study in AIDS research has resulted in the suggestion of fruitful questions for research based on the personal experiences of women being ignored. In addition to reports by women that their continuing yeast infections and pelvic inflammatory disease are not the result of noncompliance with medication (Hoegsberg et al., 1988; Carpenter and Kizirian, 1993), increasing numbers of women who are testing HIV-positive (44 percent in one study) report that they cannot identify a risk factor associated with their source of infection (Ward et al., 1988). Statements by women that their only possible risk behavior might have been heterosexual intercourse with a male who had told them he was not HIV-positive were not taken seriously by most researchers until they were corroborated by a study of *men* in which 35 percent admitted that they would lie to a potential sex partner about their HIV status, and 20 percent said they had lied about having been tested (Elkin, 1990). In a similar vein, much of the education and advertising campaigns about condom use have been directed toward women, despite reports by some women that requiring condom use increases battering by their partners (Anastos and Marte, 1989). Virtually none of the literature in clinical research or the information given to health care practitioners addresses the complications with their own AIDS illness that women face because they may also be the caretaker of a male partner or child who has the disease.

APPROACHES AND METHODS

Male-centered approaches to the definition and choice of problems for study have led to experimental approaches and methods which tend to exclude women as experimental subjects and to ignore pertinent issues in women's health. Considerable attention (Wheeler, 1990) has been drawn to the failure of the National Institutes of Health (NIH) to include female research subjects. Under pressure from Congress, NIH has set up a new Office of Research on Women's Health to ensure that women's health needs are addressed and to enforce their policy of including women in their research unless it involves a disease that affects only men (Pinn and LaRosa, 1992).

Drug testing in AIDS provides a clear-cut example of this failure to include women as experimental subjects. Most of the drug trials have specifically excluded women. The original studies of AZT, the most frequently prescribed drug in AIDS treatment, despite recent controversy (GayNet News Service, 1993) surrounding its effectiveness, included only 13 women out of 282 patients (Fischl et al., 1987). Only after considerable protest and public attention were directed toward this exclusionary behavior did women begin to be routinely included. A national study of AZT called Protocol 076 sought 700 pregnant women to determine if the drug reduces the chance of an infected woman's transmitting the virus to the baby. The study originally included no maternal health component. Although pregnant women were eventually included, it was "not for purposes of the woman's health" (Byron, 1991, p. 26). An AIDS clinical trial group study of pentamidine, dapsone, and zidovudine excluded "pregnant and lactating women and women of childbearing potential" (National Institute of Allergy and Infectious Diseases, as quoted in Anastos and Marte, 1989).

Using only males as experimental subjects ignores the fact that females may respond differently to the drug being tested, and it may lead to less accurate models even in the male (Hoffman, 1982). A reported effect of AIDS in women is changes in the menstrual cycle and pregnancy (Marte and Anastos, 1990), which may indicate changes in the normal hormone levels. Given the numerous opportunistic infections and depression in the immune system of AIDS patients, it would not be surprising to find fluctuations in hormone levels of male AIDS victims. Furthermore, testing of drugs in pregnant female rats and other lower animals is a first step toward discovering the effects of treatment drugs on the developing fetus. These baseline studies in female animals, including pregnant females, are imperative for establishing baseline data for testing in humans.

When women subjects have been included in research on the epidemiology and progression of AIDS or in experimental drug trials, often they have been treated as less than human. Sometimes the emphasis is on women as vectors for transmission rather than as sick people themselves.

The high incidence (51 percent) of AIDS resulting from IV drug use in women (Anastos and Marte, 1989) is used as a justification for poor funding for research and treatment for women with AIDS. IV drug use does represent a risk behavior that is difficult to control without massive funds for treatment and education. However, women have a higher rate of "undetermined means of acquiring infection" (9 percent) compared to men (2 percent) (Anastos and Marte, 1989). The group of women at double risk from infection as IV drug users and partners of infected men or men at risk is not calculated separately for women as it is routinely for men (Anastos and Marte, 1989).

Frequently it is difficult to determine whether these women are treated as less than human because of their gender or whether race and/or class are more significant variables. AIDS infection in minority women occurs at a much higher rate than their proportion in the overall population or than the rate of AIDS infection in white women (Willoughby, 1989). Class also is a significant risk factor for AIDS. When researchers examined New York City data by zip code, they discovered that the most socially and economically devastated inner-city areas are those with the most HIV disease (NYC Community Health Atlas, 1988; Kolata, 1993). A 1993 National Research Council Study found that AIDS was heavily concentrated in six to ten neighborhoods in New York City (Kolata, 1993). Women who are both poor and Black or Hispanic may face double discrimination because of both race and class.

In *And the Band Played On*, Shilts (1987) critiques the health care establishment and the federal government for its negligence in responding to AIDS. Shilts proposes that because AIDS was initially discovered in the gay male population in the United States, government and health care officials were able to distance themselves from AIDS sufferers. It was functional for them to view the AIDS patients as very different from themselves, less than human, because this view protected them from the awful truth that they too might fall prey to this disease. Perhaps some of the accounts by women infected with AIDS of their inhumane treatment by being forced to abort against their will are comprehensible when viewed in this light (Marte and Anastos, 1990; Chavkin, 1989). A woman who is an IV drug user, poor, and Black is likely to differ markedly from the white male physician who may provide clinical diagnosis of her AIDS. To him she may seem so different that she is not worthy of the rights accorded all human beings about reproductive choice. Similar recent suggestions (Kolata, 1993) that AIDS may be contained because it occurs in socially marginalized groups implies a significant difference and distance between researchers and patients.

Initial investigations of AIDS were inhibited by overreliance on the methods of one field—epidemiology. The reliance of epidemiology on population statistics led to the categorizion of AIDS by groups of people rather than risk behaviors. As soon as it became clear that certain behaviors placed an individual at risk for transmission of the virus, professionals began to recognize that interdisciplinary methods would be necessary to understand the etiology, transmission, progression, and control of the disease. Interactive models which draw on both the social and natural sciences, such as Hamilton (1985) has called for to understand health problems like heart disease, are being developed to examine AIDS. However, androcentric bias may constrict the scope of interdisciplinary methods so that they fail to integrate approaches most likely to be fruitful for understanding and combatting AIDS in women. For example, failure to include obstetricians/gynecologists and the information they are uncovering about reproductive-tract infections and diseases in HIV-positive women is a serious omission. Failure to study the impact of the crack epidemic and its associated hypersexuality in crack houses—where many women and adolescent girls exchange sex for drugs with men, many of whom may be older, IV drug users—will provide incomplete information about heterosexual transmission from men to women. Studies of crack houses using the traditional androcentric approach of viewing such women as prostitutes who are vectors for transmission to men are likely to overlook important information on AIDS in women.

THEORIES AND CONCLUSIONS DRAWN FROM THE RESEARCH

Not surprisingly, androcentric bias in the choice and definition of problems for study and methods which exclude women as experimental subjects and approaches most pertinent to women's health, result in conclusions and theories drawn from the research that also exclude women. For human-centered or patient-centered research, theories and conclusions that include people of both genders and all races, classes, ages, and sexual orientations, the research must be conceived without bias and carried out using inclusive methods. In the interim, as those biases are being corrected, information about women gleaned from current AIDS research needs to be reflected in the theories and conclusions drawn from the data.

Androcentric language should not permeate case definitions used for diagnosis, literature reports of research, or designation of individuals at risk for the disease. Revision of the CDC surveillance case definition to include unusual persistence and incidence of female reproductive-tract infections and cancers as possible indicators of AIDS in women, along with candidiasis in orifices and organs other than the vagina, provided health care professionals with a necessary tool to correct underdiagnosis of AIDS in women.

Researchers should use terms such as "prostitute" with caution. Often the important fact for AIDS research is that a woman has multiple sex partners or is an IV drug user rather than that she received money for sex. Such terms as "prostitute" may induce androcentric bias in that they promote thinking of the women as vectors for transmission to men. In fact the men may have an equal or greater number of sex partners to whom they are transmitting the disease. Even more important, by emphasizing AIDS in "prostitutes," health care practitioners are able to distance themselves and their female patients from the risk of AIDS. This may lead to practitioners' treating prostitutes as less than human and underdiagnosing AIDS in women who are not prostitutes. Focus on group characteristics such as prostitute, poor, Black, or unmarried repeats the initial mistake of identifying the disease by group rather than by behavioral risk.

Theories and conclusions drawn from AIDS research should be examined to determine to what extent they represent and reinforce the social status quo of sexism, racism, and classism harmful to women in our society. Overexamination of prostitutes and pregnant women perpetuates the madonna/whore images as the only available roles for women in our society. Targeting women for educational campaigns for AIDS prevention through condom use, without studying the risks from battering and male attitudes toward condom use, ignores the power and behavioral differences for men and women in heterosexual intercourse. It may also ignore deeply entrenched religious and cultural biases of some ethnic groups toward contraceptive use in general and condom use in particular. Testing, without informed consent, all pregnant women who obtain health care through a public health clinic further dehumanizes women, who suffer in an economy in which the average woman earns seventy-one cents for every dollar the average man earns (Green, 1990) and where 74 percent of men default on child support after divorce (Rix, 1989). Suggesting that only marginalized social outcasts are infected with AIDS (Kolata, 1993) feeds racial and class stereotypes while encouraging risky behaviors.

Uncritical acceptance of sexism, racism, and classism in our society and the consequent incorporation of those biases into AIDS research has led to the current underdiagnosis of AIDS in women and the accompanying failure to understand the disease's progression, complications, treatment, and complex transmission patterns. Researchers and practitioners who think higher absolute numbers of male individuals with AIDS or a history of accumulated baseline data in males warrants continued androcentric focus in AIDS research are being short-sighted. Aside from the ethical, moral, and legal problems raised by accepting androcentric bias once it has been revealed, researchers must correct the bias in order to help men and children, as well as women.

In the beginning, women were a focal point as caregivers in the AIDS epidemic. Eventually attention was given to women as vectors for transmission to men and children. Now is the time to shift the focus to the women themselves as human beings with the disease. Research on AIDS from a female-centered perspective will help to complete the AIDS picture for us all.

REFERENCES

Anastos, K., and Marte, C. 1989. Women—the missing persons in the AIDS epidemic. *Health/PAC Bulletin* 19, no. 4:6–13.

Birke, Lynda. 1986. *Women, feminism, and biology.* New York: Methuen.

Bleier, Ruth. 1984. *Science and gender: A critique of biology and its theories on women.* New York: Pergamon Press.

Byron, P. 1991. HIV: The national scandal. *Ms.* 1, no. 4:24–29.

Carpenter, C. C. J., and Kizirian, J. 1993. HIV infection in North American women. Abstract from First Annual Women's Health Conference. *Journal of Women's Health* 2, no. 2:204.

Centers for Disease Control. 1987. Antibody to human immunodeficiency virus in female prostitutes. *Morbidity and Mortality Weekly Report* 36:157–161.

———. 1987. Revision of the CDC surveillance case definition for acquired immunodeficiency syndrome. *Morbidity and Mortality Weekly Report* 36 (suppl.):1s-15s.

———. 1988. Distribution of AIDS cases by racial/ethnic group and exposure category, June 1, 1981–July 4, 1988. *Morbidity and Mortality Weekly Report* 37, no. SS-3:1–3.

———. 1990. AIDS among U.S. women. *Morbidity and Mortality Weekly Report.* Chart given in *Charlotte Observer,* December 1, p. 1A.

Chavkin, W.; Driver, C.; and Forman, P. 1989. The crisis in New York City's perinatal services. *New York State Journal of Medicine,* 89, no. 12:658–663.

Chavkin, Wendy. 1989. Help, don't jail, addicted mothers. *New York Times,* July 18, p. A-1.

Cohen, J., et al. 1988. Prostitutes and AIDS: Public policy issues. *AIDS and Public Policy Journal* 3:16–22.

Corea, G., et al. (eds.). 1987. *Man-made women: How new reproductive technologies affect women.* Bloomington: Indiana University Press.

Ehrenreich, Barbara, and English, Deirdre. 1978. *For her own good.* New York: Anchor Press.

Elkin, S. 1990. Information presented at session on Women and AIDS at 4th International Interdisciplinary Congress on Women. Hunter College, New York, June.

Fausto-Sterling, A. 1985; revised 1992. *Myths of gender: Biological theories about women and men.* New York: Basic Books.

Fischl, M. A., et al. 1987. The efficacy of Azidothymidine (AZT) in the treatment of patients with AIDS and AIDS-related complex: A double-blind placebo-controlled trial. *New England Journal of Medicine* 317:185–191.

GayNet News Service. 1993. No breakthroughs at AIDS conference. *Outlines* 7, no. 2 (July):10.

Gillespie, M. A. 1991. HIV: The global crisis. *Ms.* 1, no. 4:16–23.

Green, C. 1990. Women closing the income gap. *The State,* September 27, p. C-1.

Guinan, M. E., and Hardy, A. 1987. Epidemiology of AIDS in women in the United States: 1981–86. *Journal of the American Medical Association* 260:1922–1929.

Hamilton, Jean. 1985. Avoiding methodological biases in gender-related research. *Women's health report of the Public Health Service Task Force on Women's Health Issues.* Washington, D.C.: U.S. Department of Health and Human Services Public Service.

Hand, I. L., et al. 1989. Newborn screening for HIV seropositivity in the South Bronx. Fifth International Conference on AIDS, Montreal, Quebec, Canada, abstract, 120.

Haraway, D. 1978. Animal sociology and a natural economy of the body politic, Part I: A political physiology of dominance; and Animal sociology and a natural economy of the body politic, Part II: The past is the contested zone: Human nature and theories of production and reproduction in primate behavior studies. *Signs: Journal of Women in Culture and Society* 4, no. 1:21–60.

Healy, Bernadine. 1991. The Yentl syndrome. *The New England Journal of Medicine* 325, no. 4:274–276.

Hoegsberg, B., et al. 1988. *Human immunodeficiency virus in women with pelvic inflammatory disease.* The Fourth International Conference on AIDS, Stockholm, Sweden, abstract, 333.

Hoffman, J. C. 1982. Biorhythms in human reproduction: The not-so-steady states. *Signs: Journal of Women in Culture and Society* 7, no. 4:829–844.

Hubbard, Ruth. 1990. *Politics of women's biology.* New Brunswick, N.J.: Rutgers University Press.

Keller, E. 1985. Dynamic autonomy. In *Reflections on gender and science.* New Haven: Yale University Press.

Keller, Evelyn. 1983. *A feeling for the organism: The life and work of Barbara McClintock.* New York: W. H. Freeman and Company.

Kirschstein, R. L. 1985. *Women's health: Report of the Public Health Service Task Force on Women's Health Issues.* Vol. 2. Washington, D.C.: U.S. Department of Health and Human Services Public Health Service.

Kolata, Gina. 1993. Targeting urged in attack on AIDS. *The New York Times,* March 7, pp. A-1, A-26.

Livingston, Miles. 1993. Revised AIDS definition cited in rising SC cases. *The State,* May 4, p. B-1.

Marte, C., and Anastos, K. 1990. Women—the missing persons in the AIDS epidemic: Part II. *Health/PAC Bulletin* 20, no. 1:11–23.

McClintock, B. 1950. The origin and behavior of mutable loci in maize. *Proceedings of the National Academy of Sciences* 36:344–355.

Minkoff, H.; Moreno, Jonathan; and Powderly, Kathleen. 1992. Fetal protection and women's access to clinical trials. *Journal of Women's Health* 1, no. 2:137–140.

Mondanaro, J. 1987. Strategies for AIDS prevention: Motivating health behavior in drug dependent women. *Journal of Psychoactive Drugs* 19, no. 2:143–149.

Nanney, D. L. 1957. The role of cytoplasm in heredity. In W. E. McElroy and H. B. Glenn (eds.), *The chemical basis of heredity,* pp. 134–166. Baltimore: Johns Hopkins University Press.

National News Roundup. 1993. AIDS no. 1 killer of young men in 5 states, 64 cities. *Outlines* 7, no. 2(July):12.

New York City Community Health Atlas. 1988. New York: United Hospital Fund.

Norwood, C. 1988. Women and the "hidden" AIDS epidemic. *Network News,* Newsletter of the National Women's Health Network, November/December, pp. 1, 6.

Pinn, Vivian, and LaRosa, Judith. 1992. *Overview: Office of research on women's health* (October). Bethesda, Md.: National Institutes of Health.

Provenchar, D., et al. 1988. HIV status and positive Papanicolaou screening: Identification of high-risk population. *Gynecologic Oncology* 31:184–190.

Rhoads, J. L., et al. 1987. Chronic vaginal candidiasis in women with human immunodeficiency virus infection. *Journal of the American Medical Association* 257:3105–3107.

Rix, S. 1989. *The American woman, 1988–89: A status report.* New York: Norton.

Rosenberg, M. J., and Weiner, J. M. 1988. Prostitutes and AIDS: A health department priority? *American Journal of Public Health* 78, no. 4:418–423.

Rosser, S. V. 1989. Re-visioning clinical research: Gender and the ethics of experimental design. *Hypatia* 4, no. 2:125–139.

Sayre, Ann. 1975. *Rosalind Franklin and DNA.* New York: W. W. Norton and Company, Inc.

Schrager, L. K., et al. 1989. Cervical and vaginal squamous cell abnormalities in women infected with human immunodeficiency virus. *Journal of Acquired Immunodeficiency Syndrome* 2:570–575.

Selwyn, P. A., et al. 1989. Prospective study of human immunodeficiency virus infection and pregnancy outcomes in intravenous drug users. *Journal of the American Medical Association* 261:1289–1294.

Shilts, R. 1987. *And the band played on: Politics, people and the AIDS epidemic.* New York: St. Martin's Press.

The State. 1993. New definition pushes up number of AIDS cases. April 30, p. A-3.

Thomas, Lewis. 1974. *The lives of a cell.* New York: Viking.

Ward, J. W., et al. 1988. Epidemiologic characteristics of blood donors with antibody to human immunodeficiency virus. *Transfusion* 28:298–301.

Watson, James D. 1969. *The double helix.* New York: Atheneum Publishers, Mentor.

Wheeler, D. L. 1990. NIH to require researchers to include women in studies. *The Chronicle of Higher Education* 37, no. 3:A-32–33.

Willoughby, A. 1989. AIDS in women: Epidemiology. *Clinical Obstetrics and Gynecology* 32, no. 3:429–436.

World Health Organization Global Programme on AIDS. 1990. World AIDS Day 1990: Focus on women and AIDS. *World AIDS Day Newsletter* 1 (June/July):1–2.

Zuckerman, C., and Gordon, L. 1988. Meeting the psychosocial and legal needs of women with AIDS and their families. *New York State Journal of Medicine* (December):619–620.

CHAPTER THREE

Androcentric Bias in Psychiatric Diagnosis

A pivotal factor in the practice of modern psychiatry is psychiatric diagnosis. The therapist-client relationship, the suggested prognosis and treatment, and whether or not insurance will partially or completely reimburse the expenses incurred depend substantially upon psychiatric diagnosis. Flaws, biases, and ethical problems surrounding diagnosis may lead to inappropriate or inequitable treatments that exacerbate or fail to improve the misery that some individuals face as a result of their psychiatric conditions. This chapter explores some of the ways in which androcentric bias may currently affect psychiatric diagnosis, which in turn may influence the psychiatrist-patient relationship and lead to treatments which are less helpful, particularly for female clients. Some attempts to correct this androcentric focus which have been and continue to be developed by feminists are also discussed.

As a branch of clinical medicine, psychiatry has its basis in science. Freud (1968, p. 181) went to considerable effort to emphasize the scientific foundation of his psychoanalytic theory. Although he saw sexuality as the motivating and driving force within each individual and between and among individuals, he rooted the source of sexuality in biology. "Anatomy is destiny" (Freud, 1968, p. 181) has frequently been interpreted as a form of biological determinism.

BASIC SCIENCE RESEARCH

In the neurosciences, a substantial amount of work has been done relating to sex differences in the brains of men and women. As Birke (1986) and Bleier (1984) have stressed, the voluminous research on sex differences, which is well funded by federal and foundation sources and attracts considerable attention, clearly plays a significant role in our society. Numerous studies have documented (Maccoby and Jacklin, 1974) that similarities and overlaps rather than differences and clear separation between the sexes are the reality for most abilities and behaviors studied. Even in the four areas of aggression and verbal, visuo-spatial, and mathematical ability, in which studies have found differences between the sexes (Maccoby and Jacklin, 1974), those differences were statistically significant only when very large numbers were used for the sample size. The ranges between the two sexes for even these four areas overlap so much that thousands of people must be sampled to show a significant difference between the male and female means for those abilities and behaviors.

With regard to nonbiological factors such as pay inequities, child-care responsibilities, and single-parent households, there are clear separations between the sexes. Statistically significant mean differences can be easily established even when small sample sizes are used. The average female worker earns no more than seventy-one cents for every dollar earned by a male worker—a significant and clear-cut difference. Does the search for biologically based sex differences (and racial differences) represent an attempt to find biological bases for the social inequality between the sexes? One can imagine that a society free from such inequality would not view sex differences research as a valid scientific endeavor. For example, how much money and emphasis are placed upon research on differences in eye color or hair color? The fact that our society supports research on sex and racial differences indicates the extent to which the values of the society and the scientists influence the choice of topics chosen for study and the "objectivity" with which such research is likely to be approached.

Bleier (1979), Star (1979), and Sayers (1982) have critiqued the studies on brain lateralization, hormones, and brain anatomy (Bleier, 1984) that attempt to link differences in male and female brains with behavioral traits such as visuo-spatial ability, verbal ability, and aggression. These feminists have demonstrated flaws in experimental design, assumptions based on limited experimental data, unwarranted extrapolation of data from rodents to humans, and problems with biochemical conversion of hormones from estrogens to androgens within the body (Bleier, 1984). Fennema and Sherman (1977), Sherman (1980), Haven (1972), and Kelly, Whyte, and Smail (1984) have documented that social factors such as number of mathematics courses taken, familiarity with games that develop visuo-spatial skills (Caplan, MacPherson, and Tobin, 1985), and peer pressure have an extremely important effect on the differential performance of adolescent males and females on tests of mathematical ability. Feminists (Hubbard and Lowe, 1979) as well as other scientists (Lewontin, Rose, and Kamin, 1984) have pointed out the cultural and gender biases in the I.Q. test.

Feminist critiques have revealed that in their search for biological differences that may correlate well with or be used to explain differences in social, political, or economic positions between the sexes, some researchers have allowed flaws to infect their research. One such flaw is having weaker criteria for acceptance of studies providing biological evidence that can be interpreted to support the social status quo. Bleier

(1988) recounts her dealings with *Science,* a very reputable journal, over her refutation of a study it published (Utamsing and Holloway, 1982) based on the autopsy of fourteen human brains (nine male, five female). The study purported to demonstrate a sex difference in the size of the splenium of the corpus callosum between male and female brains, which would support the theory of less lateralization of the human female brain. Bleier's letters to the editor questioning the small sample size, the use of selected brains from autopsied patients without specifying age, cause of death, or mode of selection, and assumption without evidence that size of splenium reflects number of axons and degree of hemispheric lateralization were not published. Bleier's own study undertaken to refute Utamsing and Holloway, involving thirty-nine subjects (twenty-two female, seventeen male), was not sent out for review by the editor of *Science.* It was ultimately published in another journal (Bleier, Houston, and Byne, 1986).

Ironically, in their eagerness to explore sex differences, many researchers have overlooked another flaw, failure to consider *species* differences. Bleier (1984) describes the differences between the nervous system and developmental stages in the rodent and human. Just as it is not appropriate for sociobiologists to extrapolate from one species to another and generalize beyond the limits of the data on the organismal level, such extrapolations and generalizations are equally inappropriate when discussing the development of the nervous system. Although exposure to fetal androgens in the male rat prevents cyclic release of LH in response to estrogens and progestins (the so-called organizing effect), it does not have a similar effect in guinea pigs or primates, including humans (Bleier, 1984). Estrogens will elicit an LH surge in men similar to that in women (Kulin and Reiter, 1976), and androgens do *not* suppress cyclicity, ovulation, menstruation, or pregnancy in women (or nonhuman primates) exposed to fetal androgens (Bleier, 1984). Is it valid to overlook species differences in an attempt to find sex differences within a species?

Perhaps the most pervasive flaw in the neurosciences research is excessive reductionism, with its corollary assumption that neuroanatomy or neuro-secretions can be separated from their environment. Feminist critiques of the neurosciences again rest on the same basis: Genetic, hormonal, and structural effects of the brain on behavior cannot be separated from the effects upon behavior of learning and socialization in the environment. Indeed, the two are so interrelated that the environment may actually affect the prenatal structure of the brain, which may in turn affect learning abilities. As Bleier (1984) states:

> Even though genes are involved in the embryonic differentiation of the various nerve cell types and in the spatial organization of nerve cells (neurons) within the fetal brain, the final form, size, and connections between different neurons and therefore the brain's proper functioning also depend on maternal environment milieu and on input from the external world. . . . It has been

found that malnutrition throughout the period of postnatal development of rat pups results in a decrease in both the number and the size of neurons in the brain. If the pups were also malnourished in utero, they can suffer as much as a 60 percent reduction in brain cell number, as compared with controls, by the time of weaning. Human infants dying of malnutrition during the first year of life also have smaller than normal brains with a reduced number and size of neurons (Winick, 1975). (Bleier, 1984, p. 44)

ENDOCRINOLOGY

In endocrinological research, much effort has also supported the search for differences between the sexes. The terminology of "male hormones" (commonly used to describe testosterone and its derivatives) and "female hormones" (frequently used for both the estrogen-related hormones and the progestins) is a telling example of the emphasis on sex differences. In fact both of the so-called male hormones and female hormones are found in both males and females. The major difference is in the levels or amounts produced in the two sexes, not in their presence in one sex or absence in the other. There are also differences in their major anatomical sources in the adults of the two sexes (ovaries in the female, testes in the male, and adrenal glands in both males and females) and their cyclicity of production. Furthermore, there are many different forms of estrogens, progestins, and androgens, all closely related to each other in chemical structure. They all have as their basic structure the four carbon rings of cholesterol (which is the common characteristic of hormones in the class known as steroids), with the main difference among them being in one or two of the side chains having oxygen (O) or hydrogen (H). In various body tissues of both sexes, cholesterol is normally metabolized to progesterone, which is metabolized to testosterone, the major androgen, which is metabolized to estradiol, the major estrogen. There are many other circulating metabolic forms of the three steroids, each with unique physiological effects, present in varying levels in females and males, with constant conversions from some forms to others. However, use of the terms "male" and "female" hormones obscures these true differences in amount and cycle of production and suggests incorrectly to the layperson that men produce only "male hormones" and that women produce only "female hormones."

Although presumably aware of these biological subtleties regarding "male" and "female" hormones, researchers in endocrinology have produced work which suggests some fuzziness and flaws in their understanding of the relationship between hormones and sex.

Some of the work in endocrinology has assumed that the cyclical nature of the female reproductive pattern makes female rodents and primates unsuitable as experimental subjects for tests of hormones or other chemicals. Feminists in science have pointed out the problems of hormonal and drug tests, including those for human consumption

(Wheeler, 1990), run only on male subjects, which may yield "cleaner" but limited data.

This cyclicity has also led most researchers to reject the female as a model system for hormone action. The work of Hoffman (1982), however, suggests that the female body, because of its cyclic reproductive hormone levels, may provide a more accurate model for most hormones.

Because "male hormones" and "female hormones" occur in both sexes and are closely related biochemically, biochemical conversions between hormones may occur within the body. An injection of testosterone may be converted to estrogen or another derivative before it reaches the brain (Bleier, 1979). Therefore, research which purports to demonstrate that testosterone makes males more aggressive or faster at running mazes may be flawed because the testosterone injected may or may not be converted to other derivatives before it reaches the operative organs.

In addition to problems with biochemical conversions of hormones after injection, behavioral effects induced in one species do not ensure similar effects in a different species. Bleier (1979), Hubbard (1983, 1990), Lowe (1983), and Fausto-Sterling (1992) have warned repeatedly against extrapolating from one species to another with respect to biochemical traits. They also warn against the assumption that changes in hormone levels necessarily are the cause of behavioral or performance differences between the sexes.

Feminists have stressed the importance in endocrinology of the inseparability of biological and behavioral factors. Environmental physical or psychological stress factors such as position in the dominance hierarchy have been shown to be both the cause and the effect of higher or lower levels of testosterone in primates (Rose, Holaday, and Bernstein, 1971). In addition, Hrdy (1981) discusses the interrelationships between hormone levels, reproductive inhibition, and dominance in female primates.

Feminist scientists (Bleier, 1984; Birke, 1986; Fausto-Sterling, 1992) have warned against confounding the correlation of changing hormone levels and behavioral manifestations with cause and effect. This confounding is particularly likely to occur when the biological results correlate well with the social status quo.

CLINICAL RESEARCH

Psychoanalysis has come under severe criticism from diverse viewpoints (Adler, 1927; Horney, 1973; Thompson, 1964; Friedan, 1974; Deutsch, 1944; Millett, 1970) since the early part of this century. Other models of development (Erikson, 1964; Levinson et al., 1974), and other theories such as modeling (Dinnerstein, 1976), object-relations (Chodorow, 1978), learning, scripting, socialization, and power relations, are recognized now to be important components of sexuality and gender-role identity. Although these theories and others, such as behavior modification, family dynamics, and systems theories, form part of the knowledge base of the modern psychiatrist, current psychiatric practice emphasizes the biological or scientific bases of behavior.

As M.D.'s, psychiatrists differ from psychologists, counselors, and other therapists in that they have been trained more extensively in science and medicine. Their license as an M.D. permits them to prescribe drugs to change chemical and biological states that affect behavior. Psychiatrists are distinguished from other mental health professionals by their belief and grounding in scientific and medicinal approaches. The *Diagnostic and Statistical Manual of Mental Disorders* (3rd edition, revised) (DSM-III-R) represents a conscious, concerted effort to remedicalize and emphasize the biological basis for psychiatric diagnoses. The American Psychiatric Association worked closely with the group modifying the ICD-9 (*International Classification of Diseases-9*) for use in the United States to ensure that DSM-III-R "would, as much as possible, reflect the most current state of knowledge regarding mental disorders, yet maintain compatibility with ICD-9" (American Psychiatric Association, 1987, xix). The attempt to maintain compatibility with ICD-9 reinforces the medical basis for the diagnosis and reestablishes the unique position of the psychiatrist compared to other therapists. To that extent DSM-III-R represents remedicalization.

Feminists (Friedan, 1974; Millett, 1970), including feminist psychologists (Chodorow, 1978; Dinnerstein, 1977; Miller, 1976) and psychiatrists (Person, 1990), have suggested that psychiatry as one of the sciences represents a value-laden cultural enterprise. "A cultural enterprise must, by definition, be value-laden and embody a set of beliefs" (Person, 1990, p. 306). Macklin (1973) points out that in psychoanalysis, values are held by the patient and the therapist and are implicit or explicit in the theory: "As long as those values coincide, they go virtually unnoticed. Cultural biases become most apparent during times of social change, times when they no longer coincide" (Person, 1990, p. 307).

Feminists have critiqued the extent to which misogyny and androcentrism in Freudian and other theories were not revealed because they were congruent with the societal and cultural norms. These biases were also less apparent to therapists, who were predominantly male and held power over their clients, who were predominantly female and less powerful (Chesler, 1971; Gove and Tudor, 1973). "Under the impact of changing cultural norms, we have become aware of the presence of sexism in all of the psychotherapies, including psychoanalysis, and of the theoretical justifications for sexism in fundamental psychoanalytic assumptions" (Person, 1990, p. 307). Kaplan (1983a, 1983b) suggested that the various categories in DSM-III contain "masculine-biased assumptions about what behaviors are healthy and what behaviors are crazy" (p. 788). The same behaviors that are thought to indicate mental illness in a woman go unnoticed or are not perceived as unhealthy if exhibited by men. McC. Dachowski also questioned the potential male bias of the DSM-III categories:

> We are more likely to label women who cannot adapt as sick and men who cannot adapt as criminal, but in fact both groups are out of step with our social system and are being pressured, one way or another, to make significant behavioral changes if they wish to be a functioning part of our society. (1984, p. 703)

These suggestions of potential masculine bias might partially explain why women are diagnosed and treated for mental illness at a much higher rate than men (Chesler, 1972; Dohrenwend and Dohrenwend, 1976; Gove, 1979; Rohrbaugh, 1979).

To what extent does androcentric bias currently affect psychiatric diagnosis? Is there bias in the choice and definition of categories for diagnosis available in DSM-III-R? If so, how do these biases in turn influence the approaches of therapists to clients, particularly male therapists toward female clients? And finally, to what extent may androcentric bias in psychiatric diagnosis and the reflection of androcentrism in the values of the therapist lead to treatment regimens and suggestions to make clients, especially female clients, fit into roles, positions, and norms prescribed by a culture reflecting patriarchal values?

CHOICE AND DEFINITION OF DIAGNOSTIC CATEGORIES

Most of the major theories of development were originally elaborated by men (Freud, 1968; Erikson, 1964; Inhelder and Piaget, 1958; Kohlberg, 1966, 1976). Other theories, such as object-relations, learning, behavior modification, family dynamics, and systems theory, were developed by men and were frequently based on male subjects only. Although feminists (Chodorow, 1982; Miller, 1976) have challenged the potential male bias of these theories and are creating female models of development (Gilligan, 1982; Miller, 1976), and learning (Belenkey et al., 1986), the theoretical bases for most diagnostic categories were elaborated by men.

Most therapists and psychiatrists are still men. More specifically for the DSM-III-R, only two of thirteen (two of fifteen if staff liaisons are counted) of the Work Group to Revise DSM-III were women. Two of nine members of the Ad Hoc Committee to Review DSM-III-R of the Board of Trustees and Assembly of District Branches were women (American Psychiatric Association, 1987). A similar gender distribution was represented on the advisory committees for specific diagnostic categories. What are the possible biases introduced by having an overwhelming majority of male specialists define the diagnostic categories for mental disorders based on theories created by men?

Categories defined by men based on theories developed by men are likely to produce a male or androcentric perspective of reality. What is defined as worthy of diagnosis is synonymous with what is problematic from a male point of view. Assumption of the male as the norm may lead to definition or categorization of behaviors or traits not shared by most men as a disorder or unhealthy.

The now-classic studies by Broverman et al. (1970) suggest that clinicians implicitly associated psychological maturity and mental health with stereotypical male characteristics. The clinicians identified as normal female traits the same traits they associated with psychological immaturity or dysfunctioning. The list of normal female qualities included dependency and passivity, while assertiveness and independence were seen as normal male qualities. In examining the diagnostic criteria for histrionic, dependent, and borderline personality disorders, it becomes evident that many of their criteria represent exaggerations or overlaps with normal femininity. Are these disorders defined from a male-as-norm perspective?

Assumption of the male as norm may also lead to the situation where events that occur during the normal life cycle of many women are defined as problematic or requiring medicalization. Studies by Ehrenreich and English (1978), Holmes et al. (1980), and Arms (1977) suggest that the increasing medicalization of childbirth (a normal reproductive event in the lives of many women) represents a male view and attempt to control childbirth which may have coincided with (rather than caused) improvements in infant and maternal mortality and morbidity. Some of the feminist critiques of the new reproductive technologies (Corea et al., 1987; Arditti et al., 1984; Klein, 1989) suggest that they are attempts by men to intervene in the normal female reproductive processes of ovulation, implantation, and gestation. From 70 to 90 percent of women report (Reid and Yen, 1981) that they experience some amount of premenstrual syndrome, and 60 percent (Gordon et al., 1965) to 95 percent (Oakley, 1980) report some degree of postpartum depression. Do categorizations such as Late Luteal Phase Dysphoric Disorder (commonly known as PMS) represent medicalization by men of what are normal behaviors for many women during the course of their reproductive lives?

Failure to recognize androcentric bias may also lead to inadequate information about gender differences for most diagnostic categories. Depression, agoraphobia, and eating disorders are found much more commonly among women (Chambless and Goldstein, 1980; Wooley and Wooley, 1980), while antisocial personality, substance abuse disorders, and paranoid personality disorders are found more frequently among men (Kaplan, 1983a). Many of the diagnostic categories in DSM-III-R include no sex-ratio data. Since a major premise of psychiatry is that hormonal and other chemical differences can lead to behavioral differences and disorders, sex-ratio data are vital to determine possible interactive effects due to differing hormone levels in men and women.

An additional problem related to androcentrism is underdiagnosis of some problems in women and overdiagnosis of others. Studies (Sandmaier, 1981, 1982; Tallen, 1990; Jones and Jones, 1976) have suggested that alcoholism and other substance-abuse difficulties may be underdiagnosed in women because the diagnostic criteria for the disease were described using the male as norm (Roman, 1988; Squires, 1989). Because of socially conditioned "feminine" behavior, the inability of families to "see" alcoholism in women (Winotur, 1971), and the fact that fewer women work outside the home, alcoholism in women is less likely to be diagnosed, particularly at an early stage of the disease. Difficulties such as brushes with the legal system, inability to perform in an employment environment, or loud, disruptive behavior may bring male alcoholics to circumstances where they undergo diagnosis and treatment at an early stage. Many fewer studies have been done on females with alcohol dependence (DSM-III-R, 1987, 174; Roman, 1988).

It is now known that alcohol affects women differently than it does men from the moment of ingestion. Even when consuming equal amounts of alcohol at equal intervals, women become intoxicated more rapidly than men because their bodies contain a higher percentage of fatty tissue, which intensifies the blood-alcohol concentration (Roman, 1988). In the long term, women who drink heavily tend to develop more severe health-related problems over a shorter period of time than do men; this process is referred to as "telescoping" (Finkelstein et al., 1990).

One tragic effect of this underdiagnosis and lack of study was the failure to describe Fetal Alcohol Syndrome and Fetal Alcohol Effect until 1973 (Jones et al., 1973). Beginning in Carthage and Sparta (Plant, 1985) in ancient times and repeatedly throughout history, references were made to the substantial numbers of women alcoholics who drank during pregnancy and produced babies with defects that are now associated with the syndrome. A second tragic effect has been the consequent failure to develop treatment models that work for women. The male norm of confrontation, institutionalization away from family members, and large group sessions (Tallen, 1990) is less appropriate for women who need support and cooperation to take care of their children while in treatment (Tallen, 1990).

While androcentrism may lead to underdiagnosis of some problems in women, it may lead to overdiagnosis of others. The classic example of overdiagnosis was the Freudian theoretical contention that a clitoral-to-vaginal transfer in orgasm must occur for a woman to attain true maturity and femininity. The work of Masters and Johnson (1966) revealing that all orgasms are dependent on adequate clitoral stimulation demonstrated the androcentrism of Freudian theory in its emphasis upon vaginal penetration as the source of orgasm for the mature woman. Despite this breakthrough, many women question whether similar male perspectives continue to lead to overdiagnosis of frigidity (Person, 1990) and other conditions in women because they are especially problematic for men.

Women often are ignored when they try to say what is or is not important to them based upon their personal experience. Freud's use of the single concept of penis envy to explain the development of sexuality, normal gender development, and neurotic conflict in women (Person, 1990, p. 310) was repudiated quickly by female psychoanalysts of the day. Horney (1924, 1926, 1932, 1933) challenged penis envy, ascribing femininity to female biology and awareness of the vagina, not disappointment over lacking a penis. Thompson (1950) suggested that the major sexual dilemma for women was not penis envy, but acknowledging their own sexuality in this culture. Other women (de Beauvoir, 1974) stated that what women envied was men's power, not their penis.

Although penis envy is no longer accepted as the central concept to explain the development of female sexuality, persistence of similarly androcentric views may be biasing current theories and diagnoses. For example, Shere Hite's work (1976) suggests that failure to achieve orgasm in women results from a male definition of the sexual act. Ninety-six percent of women achieve orgasm through masturbation (Hite, 1976, p. 411), while only 30 percent achieve orgasm during coitus (Hite, 1976, p. 423). Hite's survey revealed that many women enjoy "foreplay" and "afterplay" as much as or more than the "act" of orgasm. Hite suggests that these terms demonstrate a male view of sexual activities.

These four types of androcentric bias raise ethical issues. Psychiatrists must treat the majority of their patients (and of the population as a whole), who are female, based on diagnostic categories which may use a male as the standard for definition, which in turn may lead to possible underdiagnosis or overdiagnosis of specific conditions in women. The male as norm or androcentric bias may also lead to overmedicalization of events that normally occur during women's reproductive lives and to ignoring personal experiences or accounts by women themselves.

APPROACHES DURING THERAPY

Androcentric bias in psychiatric theory and its reflection in diagnostic categories may also distort approaches during therapy, particularly in the case of a male psychiatrist with a female patient. Feminists (Person, 1990; Macklin, 1973; Vaughter, 1976) have written a considerable amount regarding the extent to which the power differential between psychiatrist and patient may reinforce the powerlessness that most women experience in our society, particularly if the psychiatrist is male and the patient is female. An unethical, harmful example of this reinforcement is the male psychiatrist who engages in sexual relations with his female patient. This type of behavior is especially detrimental to a woman who has previously been raped, battered, or experienced frigidity. This example illustrates an extreme, unprofessional, and unethical reflection of androcentric bias in approach. More subtle issues arise with respect to the extent to which values held by the therapist may influence his/her applications of the categories for diagnosis and relationship with the patient.

Trained as physicians, many psychiatrists accept the premise of biological bases for behavior and mental disorders also reflected in Freudian theory and the current trend toward remedicalization of psychiatry. This value may predispose psychiatrists to favor biological causes for disorders that have social factors as a major, if not primary, cause.

Since women as a group possess less power, less money, and less prestige in our society than men as a group, it is not unreasonable to assume that some disorders, such as depression, are likely to be more common in women, partially because of social, stressful factors (Uhlenhuth et al., 1974). However, numerous studies have revealed that drugs are overprescribed to women to combat depression and prescribed for women at higher rates than for men also suffering from depression (Klerman and Weissman, 1985). Despite questions from feminists, therapists, and feminist therapists about the excessive use of drugs to silence women and keep them out of physicians' offices, since families and social conventions tolerate depressed women and alcoholic men but not depressed men and alcoholic women (Winotur et al., 1971), new studies emphasize chemical approaches to depression (Klerman and Weissman, 1985). A recent study documented that women continue to be perceived as more depressed than men and are still prescribed twice the amount of tranquilizers men are for the same psychological problems (Finkelstein et al., 1990). Drug therapies such as tricyclical antidepressants, monoamine inhibitors, and estrogens may show differing degrees of effectiveness in certain classifications of depression. However, psychiatrists, particularly male psychiatrists, may need to be reminded of the effects of marital role (Gove, 1972), life stress (Uhlenhuth et al., 1974), and women's low social status (Klerman and Weissman, 1985) as significant contributors to the higher incidence of depression in women than men.

A male psychiatrist is likely to view the world from a male perspective and to have had experiences common to most men in our culture. As a result he will be less likely to be able to see incongruities and inconsistencies between theories and categories for diagnosis and their application to his women patients. A male psychiatrist will have had the opportunity to relate to women only as a man. He may hold somewhat theoretical or idealized views about women, based upon his own interactions with wives, mothers, daughters, lovers, and female co-workers. His own lack of experience in dealing with the world as a woman may lead him to approach and diagnose patients in limited ways which reify theories and categories for diagnosis unsuitable to all women (Franks and Burtle, 1974).

In addition to the difference of gender, psychiatrists may also differ from many of their patients with regard to race, class, ethnic origin, religion, sexual orientation, or other significant characteristics. Most of the theories and diagnostic categories reflect not only a male perspective but a white, middle- to upper-class, Judaeo-Christian, heterosexual perspective as well. Since these same descriptors also typify most psychiatrists, their personal experiences may not have provided them with opportunities to recognize the bias emanating from those descriptors which becomes embedded in diagnostic categories.

A classic example of this bias is the fact that until the declaration otherwise by the American Psychological Association in 1973, homosexuality was considered a mental illness. Critiques revealed that previous categorization represented reification of perceptions of Freudian theory, and reinforcement of societal prejudice by psychiatrists against homosexuals.

The research of Belle (1984) and Belle et al. (1981) demonstrates that being poor and a member of an ethnic minority may contribute significantly to depression in women. Her work and that of other researchers (Gibbs, 1986; Makosky, 1982) reveal that inadequate housing, dangerous neighborhoods, and financial concerns are more serious stressors than acute crises and are extremely detrimental to women's mental health. Many minority women with low incomes are also immigrants in the process of adjusting to the demands of a new country with a different language and culture; they may also be single parents, struggling with several children. In short, they may share few characteristics with the white, male, married, affluent American-born psychiatrist.

Gender, class, race, and ethnic origin may have considerable influence on both men's and women's conceptions of parenthood, sex-role socialization, and sexuality in our society. Gender interacts with race, class, ethnic origin, and other variables in the definition of normal, healthy, and acceptable mental order in our society. Psychiatrists must constantly strive to reveal bias resulting from such interlocking variables in theories and diagnostic categories.

Differences in gender, race, class, ethnic origin, and sexual orientation may separate the psychiatrist from the patient. A factor which further encourages this gap is the scientific foundation of psychiatry in notions surrounding objectivity and distance between the observer and the subject of study (Keller, 1985). Neutrality and distance may be seen as substitutes for bias and value-laden approaches by some practitioners.

This encouraged distance may explain why some therapists seem to see their patients as less than human and/or to treat them in a less than humane manner. Perhaps it is easier to counsel an individual to defer her sexual satisfaction to that of her husband (seen by the psychiatrist as demanding too much sex), place her career goals second to those of her husband (seen by the therapist as seeking masculine pursuits), or abandon her children for treatment for alcoholism (seen by the psychiatrist as holding the family together) when the male psychiatrist knows he will never have to make such choices himself. To the extent that the diagnostic categories and the theories upon which they are based reflect and in turn support the patriarchy and social status quo, they may seem appropriate and morally right to the male psychiatrist who maintains considerable power from endorsing the status quo.

TREATMENT

The prescribed treatment in psychiatry is based on diagnosis. Although psychiatric treatment has always turned upon appropriate diagnosis, remedicalization of psychiatry, third-party reimbursement, and the DSM-III-R itself entrench the importance of diagnosis and diagnostic categories. Any androcentric bias here is likely to be reflected further in treatment bias.

Androcentric language or language which reflects bias about sex-appropriate behavior may be used by psychiatrists to describe, or conceptualize to themselves, the behavior of patients. An awareness of language should aid psychiatrists in avoiding the use of terms such as "tomboyism" (Money and Erhardt, 1972), "aggression," and "hysteria" which reflect assumptions about sex-appropriate behavior (Hamilton, 1985) that permeate behavioral descriptions in clinical research and may affect treatment regimens.

An androcentric view suggesting that events which are experienced by most women during the course of their reproductive lives are unhealthy or need to be controlled may be reflected in medical treatment for those events. Prescription of progestins to control premenstrual syndrome (PMS) and routine administration of hormone replacement therapy (HRT) for irritability during menopause may be examples of such treatment. Progestins for PMS and HRT for menopause may be appropriate treatments after other avenues such as changes in diet, exercise, and stress levels have been attempted. However, routinely administering drugs for these events before attempting other solutions may constitute androcentric treatment.

Use of the male norm for diagnosis and failure to adequately study the course of some disorders in women has led to treatment models which are less effective for women than for men. A treatment model which has been most accurately critiqued for androcentrism is alcoholism (Tallen, 1990; Nellis, 1980). The techniques of separation from family, confrontation of conflict, and ancillary, but different, support groups for co-dependents work for men. They are less effective for women, who often have major, if not sole, responsibility for child care, lose more self-esteem from confrontational approaches, and frequently enter treatment simultaneously with the breakup of a marriage or relationship.

Only 20 percent of treatment programs offer services to women (Yandow, 1989); even fewer of those (8 percent) offer child-care services to women with children (Finkelstein, 1990) or pregnant alcoholics. It is estimated that nine in ten men leave alcoholic wives, while only one in ten women leaves an alcoholic husband (Jacobbi, 1983). Most treatment programs also fail to address the underlying problems of rape, incest, or abuse for which women may be using alcohol as a medication to mitigate coping with the trauma (Bernard, 1990).

Treatments which encourage women to stay in abusive (or even unsatisfying) relationships, defer their needs and desires to those of their husbands and/or children, and be less aggressive in their career and sexual relationships must be examined for androcentric bias. Treatments which support the social status quo, place all responsibility and blame on the individual woman, and seek to maintain the traditional position of women in the family may suffer from such bias (Millett, 1970; Person, 1990; Brodsky, 1977). While helpful for maintaining a patriarchal society, these treatments may not be healthy for individual women.

There are several signs that steps are being taken to overcome androcentrism in psychiatric diagnosis. The reemergence of the feminist movement in the 1970s and its accompanying critiques of psychiatry along with other societal institutions have had a substantial impact upon psychiatric diagnosis. Some examples of this impact include acceptance that all orgasms in females are clitoral (Masters and Johnson, 1966), that career ambitions in women do not represent masculine urges (Lerner, 1980), and that women have the right to desire both sexual fulfillment and intimacy from their partners (Person, 1990), and the fact that lesbianism is no longer being classified as an illness. DSM-III-R reflects these changes in its diagnostic categories.

The women's movement and its legal actions also were effective in removing barriers for women's entrance into medicine, thereby providing opportunities for more women to become psychiatrists. In 1990, 42.9 percent of psychiatry residents and 50 percent of child psychiatry residents were women (Bickel and Quinnie, 1992). Women psychiatrists have one common variable—gender—with most patients. Many women psychiatrists and therapists will still differ in race, class, ethnic origin, and/or sexual orientation from their clients. However, the commonality of gender has led many women psychiatrists to identify themselves as feminists. They have been instrumental in providing new theories and direct psychotherapeutic services which do not blame the victim for problems of women such as rape (Burgess and Holmstrom, 1973), family violence (Walker, 1978), depression (Bart, 1971), and abortion. As feminists they have sought not only to critique androcentrism in psychiatric theories and diagnostic categories but also to develop approaches to clients which are less distancing, more cognizant of individual variations among women, and more humane. These critiques and approaches are encouraging treatment models and regimens more suited to the female norm and lifestyle.

The women's movement and an increase of women in the profession may have initiated changes to remove the most overt forms of androcentric bias in psychiatric diagnosis. However, many subtle evidences of androcentrism still exist. The remedicalization of psychiatry, as also evidenced in DSM-III and DSM-III-R, may lead to increased androcentrism, since medicalization in other arenas has often paralleled an increased attempt by men to control women's lives. The new diagnostic categories Late Luteal Phase Dysphoric Disorder and Self-defeating Personality Disorder proposed in DSM-III-R should be evaluated carefully by practitioners for potential androcentric bias and its consequent effects on women's lives.

I am grateful to Lebert H. Harris, M.D., and Eugene H. Kaplan, M.D., for their insightful discussions regarding this chapter, and particularly for their thoughts on the remedicalization of psychiatry.

REFERENCES

Adler, Alfred. 1927. *Understanding human nature.* New York: Greenberg.

American Psychiatric Association. 1987. *Diagnostic and statistical manual of mental disorders.* 3rd ed. revised. Washington, D.C.: APA.

Arditti, Rita, et al. 1984. *Test-tube women: What future for motherhood?* London: Pandora Press.

Arms, Suzanne. 1977. *Immaculate deception: A new look at women and childbirth in America.* New York: Bantam Books.

Bart, Pauline. 1971. Depression in middle-aged women. In V. Gornick et al. (eds.), *Women in sexist society.* New York: Basic Books.

Belenkey, Mary F., et al. 1986. *Women's ways of knowing.* New York: Basic Books.

Belle, D. 1984. Inequality and mental health: Low income and minority women. In L. Walker (ed.), *Women and mental health policy.* Newbury Park, Calif.: Sage.

Belle, D., et al. 1981. Income, mothers' mental health and family functioning in a low-income population. In American Academy of Nursing (ed.), *The impact of changing resources on health policy.* Kansas City: American Nurses Association.

Bernard, Charles. 1990. Alcoholism and sexual abuse in the family: Incest and marital rape. *Journal of Chemical Dependency* 3, no. 1:133.

Bickel, Janet, and Quinnie, Renee. 1992. *Women in medicine statistics.* Washington, D.C.: Association of American Medical Colleges.

Birke, Lynda. 1986. *Women, feminism, and biology: The feminist challenge.* New York: Methuen.

Bleier, Ruth. 1979. Social and political bias in science: An examination of animal studies and their generalizations to human behavior and evolution. In Ruth Hubbard and Marian Lowe (eds.), *Genes and gender II: Pitfalls in research on sex and gender*, pp. 49–70. New York: Gordian Press.

———. 1984. *Science and gender: A critique of biology and its theories on women.* Elmsford, N.Y.: Pergamon Press.

———. 1988. *Science* and the construction of meanings in the neurosciences. In Sue V. Rosser (ed.), *Feminism within the science and health care professions: Overcoming resistance.* Elmsford, N.Y.: Pergamon Press.

Bleier, R.; Houston, L.; and Byne, W. 1986. Can the corpus callosum predict gender, age, handedness, or cognitive differences? *Trends in Neurosciences* 9:391–394.

Brodsky, A. 1977. Countertransference issues and the woman therapist: Sex and the student therapist. *The Clinical Psychologist* 30:12–14.

Broverman, I. K., et al. 1970. Sex-role stereotypes and clinical judgments of mental health. *Journal of Consulting and Clinical Psychology* 34, no. 1:1–7.

Burgess, A., and Holmstrom, L. 1973. Rape trauma syndrome. *American Journal of Psychiatry* 131:981–986.

Caplan, P. J.; MacPherson, G. M.; and Tobin, P. 1985. Do sex-related differences in spatial abilities exist? *American Psychologist* 40:786–799.

Chambless, D., and Goldstein, A. 1980. Anxieties: Agoraphobia and hysteria. In A. Brodsky et al. (eds.), *Women and psychotherapy*. New York: Guilford.

Chesler, Phyllis. 1971. Patient and patriarch: Women in the psychotherapeutic relationship. In V. Gornick et al. (eds.), *Women in sexist society*. New York: Basic Books.

———. 1972. *Women and madness*. New York: Avon.

Chodorow, Nancy. 1978. *The reproduction of mothering*. Berkeley: University of California Press.

Corea, Gena, et al. (eds.). 1987. *Man-made women: How new reproductive technologies affect women*. Bloomington: Indiana University Press.

de Beauvoir, Simone. 1974. *The second sex*. Trans. and ed. H. M. Parshley. New York: Vintage Books.

Deutsch, Helene. 1944. *The psychology of women*. Vol. 1. New York: Greene and Stratton.

Dinnerstein, Dorothy. 1976. *The mermaid and the minotaur*. New York: Harper and Row.

Dohrenwend, B., and Dohrenwend, B. 1976. Sex differences and psychiatric disorders. *The American Journal of Sociology* 81:1447–1454.

Ehrenreich, Barbara, and English, Deirdre. 1978. *For her own good: 150 years of the experts' advice to women*. New York: Anchor Press.

Erikson, Erik. 1964. The inner and outer space: Reflections on womanhood. *Daedalus* 73, no. 2:582–606.

Fausto-Sterling, Anne. 1992. *Myths of gender*. New York: Basic Books.

Fennema, Elizabeth, and Sherman, Julia. 1977. Sex related differences in mathematics achievement, spatial visualization and affective factors. *American Educational Research Journal* 14:51–71.

Finkelstein, Norma. 1990. Treatment Issues: Women and substance abuse. Unpublished essay prepared for the National Coalition of Alcohol and Drug Dependent Women and Their Children.

Finkelstein, Norma; Duncan, Sally A.; Derman, Laura; and Smeltz, Janet. 1990. *Getting sober, getting well*. Cambridge, Mass.: Women's Alcoholism Program of CASPAR, Inc.

Franks, V., and Burtle, V. (eds.). 1974. *Women in therapy: New psychotherapies*. New York: Bruner/Mazel.

Freud, Sigmund. 1968. The passing of the Oedipus complex. In Freud, *Sexuality and the psychology of love*. New York: Collier Books.

Friedan, Betty. 1974. *The feminine mystique*. New York: Dell.

Gibbs, R. 1986. Social factors in exaggerated eating behavior among high school students. *International Journal of Eating Disorders* 5:1103–1107.

Gilligan, Carol. 1982. *In a different voice: Psychological theory and women's development*. Cambridge, Mass.: Harvard University Press.

Gordon, R. E., et al. 1965. Factors in postpartum emotional adjustment. *Obstetrics and Gynecology* 25, no. 2 (February):158–166.

Gove, W. 1979. Sex differences in the epidemiology of mental disorder: Evidence and explanations. In E. Gomberg et al. (eds.), *Gender and disordered behavior*. New York: Brunner/Mazel.

Gove, W., and Tudor, J. 1973. Adult sex roles and mental illness. *American Journal of Sociology* 73:812–835.

Gove, W. R. 1972. The relationship between sex roles, marital status, and mental illness. *Social Forces* 51, no. 1:34–44.

Halpern, D. F. 1986. *Sex differences in cognitive abilities.* Hillsdale, N.J.: Erlbaum.

Hamilton, Jean. 1985. Avoiding methodological biases in gender-related research. *Women's health report of the Public Health Service Task Force on Women's Health Issues.* Washington, D.C.: U.S. Department of Health and Human Services Public Service.

Haven, E. W. 1972. Factors associated with the selection of advanced academic mathematical courses by girls in high school. *Research Bulletin* 72:12. Princeton: Educational Testing Service.

Hite, Shere. 1976. *The Hite report: A nationwide study of female sexuality.* New York: Dell Publishing Company.

Hoffman, Joan C. 1982. Biorhythms in human reproduction: The not-so-steady states. *Signs: Journal of Women in Culture and Society* 7, no. 4:829–844.

Holmes, Helen B., et al. (eds.). 1980. *Birth control and controlling birth: Women centered perspectives.* Clifton, N.J.: The Humana Press.

Horney, Karen. 1924. On the genesis of the castration complex in women. *International Journal Psychoanalysis* 5:50–65.

———. 1926. The flight from womanhood: The masculinity-complex in women, as viewed by men and by women. *International Journal Psychoanalysis* 7:324–339.

———. 1932. The dread of women: Observations on a specific difference in the dread felt by men and by women respectively for the opposite sex. *International Journal Psychoanalysis* 13:348–360.

———. 1933. The denial of the vagina: A contribution to the problem of the genital anxieties specific to women. *International Journal Psychoanalysis* 14:57–70.

———. 1973. *Feminine psychology.* New York: Norton.

Hrdy, Sarah. 1981. *The women that never evolved.* Cambridge, Mass.: Harvard University Press.

Hubbard, Ruth. 1983. Social effects of some contemporary myths about women. In Marian Lowe and Ruth Hubbard (eds.), *Woman's nature: Rationalizations of inequality.* Elmsford, N.Y.: Pergamon Press.

———. 1990. *The politics of biology.* New Brunswick, N.J.: Rutgers University Press.

Hubbard, Ruth, and Lowe, Marian. 1979. Introduction. In Ruth Hubbard and Marian Lowe (eds.), *Genes and gender II: Pitfalls in research on sex and gender.* New York: Gordian Press.

Hyde, J. S., and Linn, M. C. (eds.) 1986. *The psychology of gender: Advances through meta-analysis.* Baltimore: Johns Hopkins.

Inhelder, B., and Piaget, J. 1958. *The growth of logical thinking from childhood to adolescence.* New York: Basic Books.

Jaccobi, Marianne. 1983. Why can't a woman drink like a man? *Boston Magazine* (March):157–161.

Jones, Ben M., and Jones, Marilyn K. 1976. Women and alcohol: Intoxication, metabolism and the menstrual cycle. In M. Greenblatt et al. (eds.), *Alcohol problems in women and children,* pp. 1030–1036. New York: Greene and Stratton.

Jones, K. L.; Smith, D. W.; Ulleland, C. N.; and Strassguth, A. P. 1973. Pattern of malformation in offspring of alcoholic mothers. *Lancet* 9:1267–1271.

Journal of the American Medical Association. 1989. Education Issue, 262, no.8:1033.

Kaplan, M. 1983a. A woman's view of DSM-III. *American Psychologist* 38:786–792.

———. 1983b. The issue of sex bias in DSM-III: Comments on the articles by Spitzer, Williams, and Kass. *American Psychologist* 38:802–803.

Keller, Evelyn. 1985. Dynamic autonomy. In *Reflections on gender and science.* New Haven: Yale University Press.

Kelly, A.; Whyte, J.; and Smail, B. 1984. *Final report of the GIST Project.* Manchester: University of Manchester, Department of Sociology.

Klein, Renate D. 1989. *Infertile women speak out about their experiences of reproductive medicine.* London: Pandora Press.

Klerman, Gerald, and Weissman, Myrna. 1985. Depressions among women. In Juanita Williams (ed.), *Psychology of women selected readings*, 2nd ed., pp. 484–513. New York: W. W. Norton and Co.

Kohlberg, L. 1966. A cognitive-developmental analysis of children's sex-role concepts and attitudes. In E. Maccoby (ed.), *The development of sex differences.* Stanford: Stanford University Press.

———. 1976. Moral stages and moralization: The cognitive-developmental approach. In T. Lickona (ed.), *Moral development and behavior.* New York: Holt, Rinehart and Winston.

Kulin, H., and Reiter, E. O. 1976. Gonadotropin and testosterone measurement after estrogen administration to adult men, prepubertal and pubertal boys, and men with hypogonadotropism. *Pediatric Research* 10:46–51.

Lerner, H. 1980. Penis envy: Alternatives in conceptualization. *Bulletin Menninger Clinic* 44:39–48.

Levinson, D. J., et al. 1974. The psychosocial development of men in early adulthood and the mid-life transition. In D. F. Ricks et al. (eds.), *Life history research in psychotherapy 3.* Minneapolis: University of Minnesota Press.

Lewontin, Richard C.; Rose, Steven; and Kamin, Leon J. 1984. *Not in our genes: Biology, ideology, and human nature.* New York: Pantheon.

Linn, M. C., and Petersen, A. C. 1985. Emergence and characterization of sex difference in spatial ability: A meta-analysis. *Child Development* 56:1479–1498.

Lowe, Marian. 1983. The dialectic of biology and culture. In Marian Lowe and Ruth Hubbard (eds.), *Woman's nature: Rationalizations of inequality.* Elmsford, N.Y.: Pergamon Press.

Maccoby, E., and Jacklin, C. 1974. *The psychology of sex differences.* Stanford, Calif.: Stanford University Press.

Macklin, R. 1973. Values in psychoanalysis and psychotherapy: A survey and analysis. *Journal American Psychoanalytic Association* 33:133–150.

Makosky, V. 1982. Sources of stress: Events or conditions? In D. Bell (ed.), *Lives in stress: Women and depression.* Newbury Park, Calif.: Sage.

Masters, William H., and Johnson, V. E. 1966. *Human sexual response.* Boston: Little, Brown.

McC. Dachowski, M. 1984. DSM-III: Sexism or societal reality? *American Psychologist* 39:702–703.

Miller, Jean B. 1976. *Toward a new psychology of women.* Boston: Beacon Press.

Millett, Kate. 1970. *Sexual politics.* Garden City, N.Y.: Doubleday.

Money, John, and Erhardt, Anke. 1972. *Man and woman, boy and girl.* Baltimore: Johns Hopkins University Press.

Nellis, Mariel. 1980. *The female fix.* Boston: Houghton-Mifflin.

Oakley, Ann. 1980. *Women confined.* New York: Schocken Books.

Person, Ethel. 1990. The influence of values in psychoanalysis: The case of female psychology. In Claudia Zanardi (ed.), *Essential papers on the psychology of women*, pp. 211–267. New York: New York University Press.

Plant, Moira. 1985. *Women, drinking, and pregnancy.* London: Tavistock Publications, Ltd.

Reid, Robert L., and Yen, S. S. 1981. Premenstrual syndrome. *American Journal of Obstetrics and Gynecology* 139:86.

Rohrbaugh, J. 1979. *Women.* New York: Basic Books.

Roman, Paul M. 1988. Biological features of a woman's alcohol use: A review. *Public Health Reports* 103, no. 6 (November/December):628–641.

Rose, R. M.; Holaday, J. W.; and Bernstein, I. S. 1971. Plasma testosterone, dominance rank, and aggressive behavior in male rhesus monkeys. *Nature* 231:366–368.

Sandmaier, Marian. 1981. *The invisible alcoholics: Women and alcohol abuse in America.* New York: McGraw-Hill Paperbacks.

———. 1982. *Helping women with alcohol problems: A guide for the community caregivers.* Philadelphia: Women's Health Communications.

Sayers, Janet. 1982. *Biological politics: Feminist and anti-feminist perspectives.* London and New York: Tavistock Publications, Ltd.

Sherman, Julie. 1980. Mathematics, spatial visualization, and related factors: Changes in girls and boys, grades 8–11. *Journal of Educational Psychology* 72:476–482.

Squires, Sally. 1989. A look at research involving women. *Washington Post,* December 27, p. WH18.

Star, Susan Leigh. 1979. Sex differences and the dichotomization of the brain: Methods, limits and problems in research on consciousness. In Ruth Hubbard and Marian Lowe (eds.), *Genes and gender II.* New York: Gordian Press.

Tallen, Bette S. 1990. Twelve step programs: A lesbian feminist critique. *NWSA Journal* 2, no. 3:390–407.

Thompson, C. 1950. Some effects of the derogatory attitude towards female sexuality. *Psychiatry* 13:349–354.

Thompson, Clara. 1964. Problems of womanhood. In M. P. Green (ed.), *Interpersonal psychoanalysis: The selected papers of Clara Thompson.* New York: Basic Books.

Uhlenhuth, E. H., et al. 1974. Symptom intensity and life stress in the city. *Archives of General Psychiatry* 31:759–764.

Utamsing, C., and Holloway, R. L. 1982. Sexual dimorphism in the human corpus callosum. *Science* 216:1431–1432.

Vaughter, R. M. 1976. Review essay on psychology. *Signs: Journal of Women in Culture and Society* 2:120–146.

Walker, L. E. 1978. Treatment alternatives for battered women. In J. R. Chapman et al. (eds.), *The victimization of women.* Beverly Hills, Calif.: Sage.

Weissman, M., and Klerman, G. 1977. Sex differences in the epidemiology of depression. *Archives of General Psychiatry* 34:98–111.

Wheeler, D. L. 1990. NIH to require researchers to include women in studies. *The Chronicle of Higher Education* 37, no. 3:A32–33.

Winick, M. 1975. Nutritional disorders during brain development. In D. B. Tower (ed.), *The clinical neurosciences.* New York: Raven Press.

Winotur, G., et al. 1971. Alcoholism IV: Is there more than one type of alcoholism? *British Journal of Psychiatry* 118:525–531.

Wooley, S., and Wooley, O. W. 1980. Eating disorders: Obesity and anorexia. In A. Brodsky et al. (eds.), *Women and psychotherapy.* New York: Guilford.

Yandow, Valery. 1989. Alcoholism in women. *Psychiatric Annals* (May):243.

CHAPTER FOUR

Separate, but Equal?

Women and Obstetrics/Gynecology

The preceding chapters have explored ways in which the domination of medicine by men may have introduced unintentional bias into research protocols, clinical trials, and treatment regimes in such widely disparate arenas as AIDS research and psychiatric diagnosis under the DSM-III-R. Male perspectives may have biased the topics and problems chosen for study, excluding those of particular significance for women's health. This exclusion may have resulted from the absence of females as experimental subjects in clinical trials, and interpretations of data extrapolated to treatments that may fail to work in the best interests of the majority of women.

Surely obstetrics and gynecology, the medical specialty that focuses specifically on women, is an area free of androcentrism, where a woman-centered or gynocentric focus thrives. By definition all the problems chosen for study are related to women's bodies and reproduction. The approaches to the issue under study must be oriented toward female anatomy, metabolism, and physiology since women and female animals must be used as experimental subjects for testing. Conclusions drawn from the data must be translated into practices appropriate to women's lives, as only women seek gynecological services.

Ironically, however, even this branch of medicine derives its norm from the heterosexual male. Obstetrics and gynecology deal primarily with issues surrounding procreation and heterosexual activity. Thus women's health care is being defined in terms of women's relationships with men. Most women first consult an obstetrician/gynecologist when they become or are thinking of becoming heterosexually active. The possibility of future problems with procreation, difficult periods, the absence of periods, or other problems surrounding menarche bring others to consult a gynecologist before they become heterosexually active. For many women, the gynecologist/obstetrician becomes the primary-care physician. Thus reproduction becomes a major focus for health care and health care research.

BASIC SCIENCE

The dual themes of male control and the male as norm emerge in the language and theories of endocrinology and development, the basic science fields in which the clinical specialty of obstetrics/gynecology is rooted. Androcentric notions about masculine and feminine gender roles also dominate the language and conceptualization of the theories used to describe reproduction and development.

Historians and philosophers of science (Haraway, 1978; Harding, 1986; Merchant, 1979; Fee, 1981, 1982; Keller, 1985) have examined the ways in which the modern mechanistic notion of science has come to represent a masculine approach to the world whereby men are given the authority to dominate and control both women and nature. In her provocative essay "The Weaker Seed: The Sexist Bias of Reproductive Theory," Nancy Tuana (1988) traces the influence of the bias of women's inferiority upon theories of human reproduction back through the preformationists to Aristotle. She argues that "adherence to a belief in the inferiority of the female creative principle biased scientific perception of the nature of woman's role in human generation" (p. 147), thereby illustrating ways in which the gender/science system informs the process of scientific investigation.

Of course, scientists today recognize numerous flaws in Aristotle's biology. Certainly his ideas that women are colder than men and therefore less developed and that women are "not the parent, just a nurse to a seed" (Aeschylus, 1975, pp. 666–669) are not acceptable to modern biologists. However, his ideas about woman's inferiority and man's providing the form and motion of the fetus were not only perpetuated in one form or another until the eleventh century, they also influenced the notion of preformation. While looking at "systematic animalcules" under the microscope, Leeuwenhoek claimed to observe two kinds of spermatozoa, one from which the male developed and the other from which the female developed (Tuana, 1988, p. 165). Clearly an example of androcentric bias influencing observation, Leeuwenhoek's "seeing" the preformed homunculus in the sperm makes sense in light of the basic belief in the primacy of the male and his active role in reproduction, which fit with social stereotypes regarding the passivity and inferiority of women for the previous two thousand years.

Feminist developmental biologists writing today (Fausto-Sterling, 1985, 1992; Biology and Gender Study Group, 1988) suggest that these same stereotypes may influence current reproductive and developmental theories. As early as 1948, Ruth Herschberger wrote a most amusing account of fertilization. By reversing the sexes, she drew attention to the extreme activity and importance assigned to the sperm as contrasted with the passivity and insignificance attributed to the role of the egg in fertilization. Emily Martin (1991) reviews the language that science has used to describe fertilization in "The Egg and the Sperm: How Science Has Constructed a Romance Based on Stereotypical Male-Female Roles."

The Biology and Gender Study Group (1988, pp. 174–175) describe the typical courtship narratives used to describe fertilization:

> Courtship is only one of the narrative structures used to describe fertilization. Indeed, "sperm tales" make a fascinating subgenre of science fiction. One of the major classes of sperm stories portrays the sperm as a heroic victor. In these narratives, the egg doesn't choose a suitor. Rather the egg is the passive prize awarded to the victor. This epic of heroic sperm struggling against the hostile uterus is the account of fertilization usually seen in contemporary introductory biology texts. The following is from one of this decade's best introductory textbooks. "Immediately, the question of the fertile life of the sperm in the reproductive tract becomes apparent. We have said that one ejaculation releases about 100 million sperm into the vagina. Conditions in the vagina are very inhospitable to sperm, and vast numbers are killed before they have a chance to pass into the cervix. Millions of others die or become infertile in the uterus or oviducts, and millions more go up the wrong oviduct or never find their way into an oviduct at all. The journey to the upper portion of the oviducts is an extremely long and hazardous one for objects so tiny. . . . Only one of the millions of sperm cells released into the vagina actually penetrates the egg cell and fertilizes it. As soon as that one cell has fertilized the egg, the [egg] cell membrane becomes impenetrable to other sperm cells, which soon die." (Keeton 1976, p. 394)

Countering the stereotype of the passive egg, Gerald and Heide Schatten (1983) have reevaluated old data and uncovered new data demonstrating a much more active role for the egg:

> In the past years, investigations of the curious cone that Wilson recorded have led to a new view of the roles that sperm and egg play in their dramatic meeting. The classic account, current for centuries, has emphasized the sperm's performance and relegated to the egg the supporting role of Sleeping Beauty—a dormant bride awaiting her mate's magic kiss, which instills the spirit that brings her to life. The egg is central to this drama, to be sure, but it is as passive a character as the Grimm brothers' princess. Now, it is becoming clear that the egg is not merely a large yolk-filled sphere into which the sperm burrow to endow new life. Rather, recent research suggests the almost heretical view that sperm and egg are mutually active partners. (p. 29)

The work of the Schattens (1983) and other investigators (Biology and Gender Study Group, 1988) has also demonstrated that the female reproductive tract is more than a passive tube through which the sperm passes in its quest for the egg. Instead, new research reveals that secretions of the female reproductive tract capacitate sperm, thus making them capable of fertilizing the egg, and activate sperm enzymes which then permit the sperm to reach the egg nucleus. This new research documents a much more active and mutual role for the female in fertilization.

Androcentrism in the form of dominance, control, and male activity pervades other aspects of developmental biology theory besides fertilization. Traditional theories of mammalian sex determination have assigned a passive role to the development of the female body condition. Using the experiments by Jost (1947, 1958) with rabbits as the prototype, they assumed that a female body type would develop in the absence of the active production of testosterone in the male. It should be noted that this theory suffered not only from extrapolation from one species to others but also from extrapolation from the generation of accessory and secondary characteristics (the experiments performed by Jost) back to primary sex determination (differentiation into ovaries or testes). This theory also *assumed* passivity in female development rather than *testing* for it. Since the development of both the male and female fetus occurs inside a pregnant female's body, it was impossible to distinguish the potential effects of the hormones from the fetal ovaries from the effects of maternal hormones produced during pregnancy.

Scientists have also critiqued more recent research on the H-Y antigen model that explains the development of testes by proposing that males synthesize a factor absent in female cells.

> Some investigators have over-emphasized the hypothesis that the Y chromosome is involved in testis determination by presenting the induction of testicular tissue as an active (gene directed, dominant) event while presenting the induction of ovarian tissue as a passive (automatic) event. Certainly, the induction of ovarian tissue is as much an active, genetically directed developmental process as is the induction of testicular tissue or, for that matter, the induction of any cellular differentiation process. Almost nothing has been written about genes involved in the induction of ovarian tissue from the undifferentiated gonad. The genetics of testis determination is easier to study because human individuals with a Y chromosome and no testicular tissue or with no Y chromosome and testicular tissue, are relatively easy to identify. Nevertheless, speculation on the kind of gonadal tissue that would develop in an XX individual if ovarian tissue induction fails could provide criteria for identifying affected individuals and thus lead to the discovery of ovarian determination genes. (Eicher and Washburn, 1986, p. 328)

Masculine and feminine social roles may have subtly pervaded other theories of developmental biology. The Biology and Gender Study Group (1988) show how theories about the relationship between the nucleus and the cytoplasm within the cell have been patterned upon husband-wife interactions within the nuclear family. The issue was who had control, the husband (nucleus) or wife (cytoplasm)—or was mutual interaction possible? "The nucleus came to be seen as the masculine ruler of the cell, the stable yet dynamic inheritance from former generations, the unmoved

mover, the mind of the cell. The cytoplasm became the feminine body of
the cell, the fluid, changeable, changing partner of the marriage" (Biology
and Gender Study Group, 1988, p. 179). The nucleus/husband and cyto-
plasm/wife analogy demonstrates the influence of gender and control on
theories of basic science. In clinical research for obstetrics/gynecology, it
is not surprising to see these influences reflected throughout the process.

CLINICAL MEDICINE

CHOICE AND DEFINITION OF PROBLEMS FOR STUDY

Clinical research in obstetrics and gynecology focuses on the female
body and the topics and problems surrounding sexual activity and reproduction. This is not a specialty in which women's bodies are overlooked
or their health issues are ignored. Amazingly, though, androcentrism still
influences the choice and definition of problems for study in different but
significant ways than in other specialties.

Women's bodies in obstetrics/gynecology serve directly as the norm
for drug testing and the standard for determining whether a topic merits
research and funding. In an indirect sense, however, this specialty derives
its norm from the heterosexual male. Because procreation and heterosexual activity constitute the major topics of research interest and the most
common reason for women to consult with an obstetrician/ gynecologist,
women's health tends to be defined in terms of relationships with men.

For most women the obstetrician/gynecologist becomes the physician
seen for periodic health checkups (Wallis, 1992). This suggests that their
first professional contact for any health issue will be the gynecologist,
who initially diagnoses, refers, or treats the patient from her/his perspective. The framework of obstetrics/gynecology (a surgical specialty), with
its focus on reproduction and sexual activity with men, provides the
norms and standards for defining women's health issues.

Centering women's health in obstetrics/gynecology may lead to research agendas which concentrate on procreation and heterosexual activities particularly important to men. Significant amounts of time and
money are expended on clinical research on women's bodies in connection
with aspects of reproduction. Since women wanted and still want to have
control over their bodies and if and when they become pregnant, women
support research on contraceptives for women. In the wake of the AIDS
epidemic, women are particularly eager for contraceptive devices such as
the female condom (Alexander, 1993) which prevent pregnancy while
providing women with some means for preventing the transmission of
sexually transmitted diseases.

Despite the desire and support of women for contraceptive research
that permits them to control their own bodies, some evidence suggests
that a motivating force behind contraceptive research is men's interest in

controlling women's bodies and the production of children. For years, virtually all contraceptive research was focused on the female, with the biological rationale that the male cycle of sperm production is more delicate and difficult to manipulate since sperm production occurs continuously, whereas women have produced all of their eggs at birth. Intolerable potential side effects such as "feminizing" effects of hormones in men provided other reasons for concentrating on the female.

Knowledge of the complexities of the hypothalamic-adenohypophyseal-ovarian interaction which controls the menstrual cycle and ovulation and its interruption by the contraceptive pill calls into question the relative delicacy of the male cycle in comparison to the female cycle. Documented deaths of users of the Dalkon Shield (the marketing success of which was based on misleading promotion) led to eventual discontinuance of all but two IUDs (Alexander, 1993) in the domestic market (Mintz, 1985). The Dalkon Shield fiasco (Mintz, 1985), coupled with evidence linking the pill to strokes, cardiovascular problems, and uterine cancer, reveals more than "potential" side effects for females who use contraceptives. Perhaps male researchers, aware of risks, have more interest in developing contraceptive technologies that cannot be applied to their own bodies but which still provide more control over the production of children.

Several other aspects of women's sexuality or reproduction have become a particular focus for regulation by gynecology. Increased research and technological intervention to enhance fertility in some groups of women, lack of Medicaid funding for abortion, and restricted and threatened abortion access for all women appear to be attempts to encourage women to have children, even unwanted children. Concurrently, forced or coerced sterilizations in women on welfare (Rodriguez-Trias, 1980; LaCheen, 1986), women of color (Dreifus, 1975; Vasquez-Calzada, 1973), or women with AIDS (Selwyn et al., 1989), and denial of access for lesbians and/or single women to artificial insemination restrict other women from becoming pregnant. Increasing use of Caesarean delivery, routine episiotomies, and the development of diverse technologies for use during the prenatal and childbirth processes further control childbirth. Older women face hysterectomies performed with increasing frequency (Centers for Disease Control, 1980; Pokras and Hufnagel, 1988; Kjerulff et al., 1992) even in the absence of disease or excessive bleeding, simply because the uterus has the potential to become cancerous (Taylor, 1979). Although estrogen replacement therapy has been demonstrated to help prevent osteoporosis and atherosclerosis, prevention of vaginal dryness to facilitate intercourse was the major reason (Wilson, 1966) physicians began to prescribe it for postmenopausal women.

These topics chosen for research and study in obstetrics and gynecology do represent real problems or important issues for women's health. However, one must question whether the intense focus on these subjects would exist if they did not represent issues of importance to women because of their relationships with men, and because of men's interest in controlling particular aspects of sexuality and reproduction.

Focusing on aspects of women's sexuality and reproduction in which men have an interest leads to the neglect of other issues of women's health less directly related to obstetrics and gynecology. Breast cancer and other diseases of the breast have received relatively little funding and study, despite the facts that the incidence of breast cancer has increased from 10 to 12.5 percent in the last ten years (Rennie, 1993) and that one in nine women can be expected to develop breast cancer during her lifetime (Henderson and Wender, 1991). Although a variety of factors are undoubtedly responsible for this lack of study, failure to identify the breast with a particular medical specialty constitutes a major factor. Breast cancer does not fit the traditional "territory" of obstetrics/gynecology, which is usually considered to be the part of a woman's reproductive system located below the waist—the ovaries, oviduct, uterus, vagina, urethra, and their associated glands. Although the breast is related through lactation to procreation and is often also involved in heterosexual activity, it is not part of the territory traditionally seen as the province of obstetrics/gynecology.

Eating disorders are another women's health issue that intersects with, but falls outside of, the "territory" of a particular specialty. Psychiatry, endocrinology, internal medicine, and even cardiology, as well as obstetrics/gynecology, may have significant information for the woman with an eating disorder. Excessive specialization, which forces concentration in one area and less synthesis from other areas of medicine, coupled with the failure of one specialty to "claim" eating disorders, leads to inadequate research on this important issue.

Similarly, other aspects of women's health only tangentially related to procreation and heterosexual activity have received little attention. Dysmenorrhea and the effects of exercise on alleviating cramps are one example. Failure to identify and fund separate studies of lesbian health issues usually results in lesbians' being lumped together with heterosexual women in studies of women's health issues. Combining lesbians and heterosexual women may obscure not only the true incidence but the cause of a disease (see chapter 7). In addition to cervical cancer, the likelihood of most sexually transmitted diseases, including gonorrhea, syphilis, herpes, and chlamydia, being transmitted from males to females during heterosexual activity is dramatically greater (Greenblatt and Schuman, 1993) than the likelihood of transmission through lesbian contact. Although such transmission between lesbians does occur, the incidence is minuscule compared to transmission between male homosexuals, or to male-to-female and female-to-male transmission during heterosexual activities.

In a related phenomenon, some reproductive issues for which both men and women are responsible become defined as solely or primarily "women's health issues." The relatively large number of contraceptive devices available for women compared to the number for men is striking. Because of the politicized climate surrounding fetal tissue research, abortion, and the litigation from the Dalkon Shield mistake (Pappert, 1986), major pharmaceutical companies are undertaking the development of few new contraceptives at this time. Thus women must shoulder the burden of contraception.

Infertility has also been defined primarily as a women's health issue, although recent data demonstrate that one-third of infertility problems are due to the male alone, 20 percent to both partners, and the rest to the female (Muller, 1990). Virtually all of the new reproductive technologies to combat infertility have been directed toward women. Some studies suggest that men may be the dominant partners in reproductive decisions of a couple to treat infertility (Muller, 1990). Lorber (1988) explains the growing popularity of in vitro fertilization to treat male infertility by men's interest in biological parenthood and women's willingness to carry the major physiological burden.

For some individual women, the new reproductive technologies may be liberating. They permit women to have children who cannot conceive because of blocked oviducts or who do not wish to have intercourse. However, since these technologies are often limited only to married women, to produce "perfect" offspring, they tend to place more control in the hands of men and the medical establishment.

APPROACHES AND METHODS

Androcentrism manifests itself somewhat differently in obstetrics/gynecology than it does in other medical specialties. Rather than excluding women as experimental subjects or overlooking or ignoring their diseases, it is reflected in excessive focus on issues directly related to procreation and heterosexual activity and which provide men with opportunities to control women's bodies. The approaches and methods of obstetric/gynecologic research also demonstrate a deflected, but pervasive, androcentric influence.

The history of obstetrics/gynecology in the United States has shown a distinct pattern of takeover and control of the childbirth and reproductive procedures (Ehrenreich and English, 1978; Holmes et al., 1980; Arms, 1977). The contest began in the nineteenth century as male physicians sought credibility and a base of economic security by wresting the control of childbirth from female midwives. The end of the nineteenth century and particularly the early part of the twentieth witnessed increasing medicalization of pregnancy, childbirth, and lactation. Concurrently there was a shift from female support and guidance during these normal reproductive events occurring in the home to male authority and control over events that were seen as requiring hospitalization and physician intervention (Harrison, 1992). Although the struggle was primarily between midwives and physicians, at various times nurses, reform-minded middle-class women, and state officials played significant roles.

By the middle of the twentieth century, the male medical establishment had gained almost complete control over childbirth in the United States and Canada, as evidenced by the fact that in 1983, 99 percent of births in the United States "occurred in hospitals, and 98 percent of these were attended by physicians" (Sullivan and Weitz, 1988, p. 1). In Canada, statistics document a similar shift in control. Although this increasing medicalization was heralded by physicians as improving the rates of infant and maternal mortality and morbidity, some evidence (Ehrenreich and English, 1978; Wertz and Wertz, 1989) suggests that these improvements were coincidental with, rather than caused by, the increasing medicalization.

The new reproductive technologies such as amniocentesis, chorionic villi biopsy, in vitro fertilization, fetal heart monitoring, and induction of labor place conception, gestation, and childbirth increasingly under medical supervision and control. Not only does each of these technologies require medical supervision for its administration, but each may also lead directly to further medical and technological intervention. For example, studies have documented that one cause for the increase in Caesarean births (from 5 percent in 1968 to 25 percent in 1987) is the use of fetal heart monitors and other current medical technologies and procedures (Boston Women's Health Book Collective, 1992). Two major investigatory studies (Marieskind, 1979; Guillemin, 1981) suggested that 33 to 75 percent of Caesareans were *not* necessary, having been performed as a result of current medical procedures and attitudes.

The availability and use of technology for each phase from conception through gestation to delivery changes the balance of power and control. Formerly conception was an event shared by a man and a woman. Pregnancy, childbirth, lactation, and postpartum constituted "normal" events in the lives of women through which they were guided by female relatives, friends, and midwives. Now the medical profession, dominated by men, controls or has the potential to control each of the phases of reproduction. This control is manifested in approaches to research which explore women-only solutions to problems of contraception and infertility or which emphasize development of new technologies, new applications of existing technologies to an increased spectrum of issues, and evaluations of technologies and their efficacy in improving fertility, pregnancy, and childbirth outcomes.

Men's increasing control of reproduction may lead to the over-medicalization of normal reproductive events in women's lives. In the preceding chapter the appropriateness was raised of a diagnosis such as Late Luteal Phase Dysphoric Disorder to label Premenstrual Syndrome (PMS), which 70 to 90 percent of women report they experience. Do this and the designation of postpartum depression, reported to some degree by

60 percent to 95 percent of women after giving birth, represent medicalization by men of normal occurrences in women's reproductive lives?

The medical profession's use of technology in menopausal and aging women further demonstrates the desire of men to control women's sexuality and reproduction. Hysterectomy is the second most common surgical procedure in the United States, (Caesarean section is first) (Kjerulff et al., 1992), performed on 550,000 women every year. This number is expected to reach 802,000 annually as baby boom women reach the age when most hysterectomies are performed (Pokras, 1989). Ninety percent of hysterectomies are performed for nonmalignant conditions such as uterine fibroids, dysfunctional bleeding, and pelvic pain (Carlson, 1991). Many gynecologists advocate hysterectomy for cancer prevention in women who have completed childbearing. Wright summed up the argument, exemplifying the focus on procreation: "The uterus has but one function: reproduction. After the last planned pregnancy, the uterus becomes a useless, bleeding, symptom-producing, potentially cancer-bearing organ and therefore should be removed" (1969, p. 560). Do doctors ever suggest removing the prostate in men since it too has the potential—much more so than the uterus—to become cancerous?

Although the advantages and disadvantages to a woman's health of hormone replacement therapy are still being explored, the pharmaceutical advertisements in medical journals appeal to physicians to use it to keep women looking young. Little study has been undertaken to evaluate alternatives to estrogen to reduce osteoporosis. The implication is that, with aging as with other aspects of women's health, women's bodies are manipulated to conform to the standards of society regarding sexuality and reproduction.

In addition to overmedicalizing normal reproductive events in women's lives, obstetrics/gynecology fails to include women whose age falls outside the range of the reproductive years. Girls and postmenopausal women remain outside the research focus. Although the health concerns of girls under fifteen and women over fifty do not rank high on the research agenda of any specialty, they are also excluded as experimental subjects from most research protocols on contraception, infertility, pregnancy, and childbirth (Minkoff, Moreno, and Powderly, 1992). One consequence of this exclusion is that very little is known about the effects of contraceptives or how to eliminate the dangers of pregnancy and childbirth should they occur in females in these very high-risk groups. Another consequence is the failure to explore secondary or even primary uses for drugs or other treatments in these age groups because the drug/treatment has been "defined" for reproductive purposes.

A prime example of such a drug is RU-486, which has been defined as an abortifacient and is used for abortions in France (Klein, Dumble, and Raymond, 1992; Chalker and Downer, 1992). Pharmaceutical companies in the United States will not undertake clinical trials with RU-486 because they fear the politically powerful pro-life lobby. Substantial evidence suggests that RU-486 is effective in treating a number of other illnesses, such as breast cancer and Cushing's syndrome, particularly prevalent in postmenopausal women. Identification of RU-486 with abortion and abortion with women of reproductive age, the subjects for obstetric/gynecologic research, leads to a prohibition on other uses for the drug for women whose ages fall outside the reproductive years.

In specialties outside of obstetrics/gynecology, women from fifteen to fifty are routinely excluded from experimental drug trials because of their reproductive capabilities. The medical establishment, pharmaceutical companies, and women themselves fear testing drugs in women who are or might become pregnant, because of teratogenic effects that might result in a deformed fetus. The tragedies caused by thalidomide and diethylstilbesterol (Direcks and Hoen, 1986) and other less well documented teratogenic effects of drugs have understandably resulted in this exclusion and caution. As a result there is little or no knowledge of the teratogenic or other effects of drugs for pregnant women approved by the FDA (Minkoff, Moreno, and Powderly, 1992). This leaves the physician and women themselves with little information upon which to base a decision about which drug could best cure or contain life-threatening illnesses with the least harm to the fetus in a pregnant patient.

Selective exclusion or inclusion of women in experimental drug trials based upon their age reveals a bias in approaches to research which provides insufficient or inaccurate information for diseases and health issues affecting some groups of women. Failure to consider the diversity among women with regard to race, class, sexual orientation, and other factors which may affect their obstetric/gynecologic health introduces additional potential biases into the research.

Recognition of the diversity among women is the first step toward defining the extent of diversity needed among experimental subjects (Minkoff, Moreno, and Powderly, 1992). A second step entails recognition that different factors of diversity may be significant for different stages of experimentation and testing. Considerable knowledge of the extent of diversity among women and how different aspects of that diversity might interact with the research in question are needed for the development of appropriate approaches.

For example, in research to develop a new contraceptive pill, women of different races (as well as ages) must be included at an early stage when biological testing of the pill is being undertaken to determine interactions and side effects with physiology, hormones, and anatomy. African-American women have a higher incidence of sickle cell anemia, fraternal twinning, and lupus erythematosus than Caucasian women. Failure to include them as subjects and to consider the interaction of the pill with these genetic and hormonal conditions might lead to disastrous, if not fatal, consequences for African-American women. Similarly, Caucasian women have a higher incidence of breast cancer than either Asian-American or African-American women. Failure to include women of diverse races in the biological testing might obscure either cancer-preventive or cancer-enhancing effects of the pill.

When the testing for the pill reaches the stage of examination for actual use, other aspects of diversity such as class, religious/ethnic affiliation, and sexual orientation may begin to emerge as significant. To some lower-income women receiving AFDC, contraceptive pills represent a further humiliation pushed on them by the government and health clinics to control their lives and "help" them decrease their government support. To many women of the Roman Catholic or fundamentalist religions, contraceptive pills may raise a conflict between religious strictures and beliefs and what the secular culture promotes as healthy and normal. To most lesbians, use of the birth control pill will be a non-issue, except when gynecologists assume a heterosexual norm (Darty and Potter, 1984) which implies that contraception will be necessary because of heterosexual intercourse. If researchers fail to consider diversity among women, along with other factors such as whether this pill helps to prevent the spread of AIDS, their approaches represent inadequate, biased testing.

Bias may also be introduced by a failure to encompass approaches from different disciplines and interdisciplinary methods. Using only the methods traditional to a particular discipline may result in limited approaches that fail to reveal sufficient information about the problem being explored. This may be a particular difficulty for research surrounding medical problems of pregnancy, childbirth, menstruation, and menopause, for which the methods of one discipline are clearly inadequate.

Methods which cross disciplinary boundaries or include combinations of methods traditionally used in separate fields may prove more appropriate. A combination of qualitative and quantitative methods may best explore varying facets of a problem. Approaches that assume that the physiological, anatomical, or other biological components are much more significant than the psychological or social factors contributing to an obstetrical/gynecological problem may lead to false results. Menstruation, ovulation, pregnancy, childbirth, lactation, and menopause all involve complex interactions between biological and psychosocial factors. Experimental approaches from a particular discipline which attempt a strict separation of these two types of factors may result in biased or very partial answers. Interactive models (Hamilton, 1985) or more holistic models (Johnson, 1992) drawn from both the social and natural sciences provide more fruitful approaches to complex problems in obstetrics/gynecology.

Researchers must not distance themselves so much from their experimental subjects that they are able to view or treat them as less than human. Approaches to experimentation that accommodate diversity among women attempt to eliminate experimental bias and provide more reliable, broadly based clinical scientific results. They must also include a commitment on the part of researchers to view all experimental subjects, regardless of their race, class, sexual orientation, or religious affiliation, as human beings entitled to the same respect and rights that they enjoy, despite their privileged position as researchers. If not, the research will not truly benefit women's health.

THE IMPACT OF RESEARCH CONCLUSIONS
ON TREATMENT AND PRACTICE

In numerous indirect, subtle ways, androcentrism in obstetrics and gynecology permeates the choice of topics and approaches to research. Not surprisingly, the influence of male control and the importance of the male perspective in defining women's health which emerge in experimental conclusions also become translated into treatment and practice.

The language obstetricians/gynecologists use to talk to their female patients, talk about them to colleagues and students, and write about the research done on them in the medical literature reflects male control and treatments prescribed for women to accommodate or satisfy their male partners. Several scholars (Benokraitis and Feagin, 1986; Association of American Medical Colleges, 1989) have investigated the language of medicine and enumerated examples which delineate different facets of the issue.

For example, many physicians routinely address women patients by their first names or use terms such as "Honey" or "Sweetie" while insisting that they be addressed as "Dr. X." This establishes authority of the physician over the patient.

When distinguishing between a partial (removal of uterus only) and total (removal of both the uterus and cervix) hysterectomy, a common joke among obstetrician/gynecologists is to describe the partial procedure as "Removing the baby box and leaving the playpen." In the "joke," the physician identifies with the male partner, for whom leaving the cervix will make sex more enjoyable. Since the cervix has few nerve endings and since most women experience uterine contractions during orgasm, removing the uterus while leaving the cervix will not usually maintain the same degree of sexual pleasure for many women.

Scientists who developed the technologies for in vitro fertilization have described women as "egg farms" and "egg factories" (Murphy, 1984). Further evidence that some scientists plan to use these technologies to control women emerges from their descriptions of a future time when, through a combination of supraovulation, in vitro fertilization, sex selection, and artificial wombs, women need be only a small percentage of the population (Postgate, 1973).

The interests of the male partner over those of the woman are also revealed in practices such as stitching up an episiotomy to make the woman "tight" for her husband (Boston Women's Health Book Collective, 1992). The episiotomy itself is a source of controversy between women and obstetricians/gynecologists in the United States. In most other countries in the world, particularly those in which midwives attend childbirth, episiotomies are rare. Even in physician-attended births outside the United States, this procedure is far from routine (Banta and Thacker, 1982). Advocates for women's health and home deliveries suggest that episiotomies routinely done in the United States represent medicalization and physicians' attempts to speed up and control the process of childbirth (Boston Women's Health Book Collective, 1992). The rationale given by obstetricians for the episiotomy is that cut tissue is easier to stitch and repair than torn tissue. Studies (e.g., Banta and Thacker, 1982) indicate, however, that episiotomies may not prevent torn tissue, damage to the baby's head, or cystocele and rectocele. Moreover, many women who do not have episiotomies experience less pain, recover faster, and have no medical complications without stitches (Kitzinger, 1981). Thus it seems that the main reason for stitches is to tighten the woman for heterosexual intercourse. A smaller vaginal opening makes the male feel like his penis fills the vagina.

Most physicians, including many women doctors, have shown cautiousness and restraint in response to the feminist health agenda. Only in limited contexts of medical care services are feminist adaptations evident. One of these is the increased availability of health-related information to women consumers, in response to the initiatives of women outside of professional circles (Ruzek, 1978). In contrast, consumers' complaints and suggestions have fostered only minor reforms in obstetrical care. The decor, ambiance, and regimens of many birthing facilities have improved to provide personal and psychological support for the mother and to promote infant-parent bonding. However, cosmetic concerns aside, efforts to increase understanding of the biology of birth and to lower infant mortality rates remain inadequate.

Further evidence of men's desire to maintain control over women's reproductive processes comes from the struggle within obstetrics/gynecology over nurse-midwives. Initiatives to use nurse-midwives as mainstream obstetric providers in the United States have met with effectively executed professional resistance. Some observers, in fact, suggest that the women's health movement has been coopted by the medical profession (Worcester and Whatley, 1988). When women started "voting with their feet" by consulting with midwives, choosing modified delivery services or hospitals with liberal labor room routines (such as admitting family members into the delivery room, not doing episiotomies, and omitting other ritualistic elements of "prep"), physicians and institutions yielded to relatively tangential demands for innovations while retaining control of the core of obstetrical care (Rothman, 1982). Establishing "the women's hospital" as a precinct within larger, existing facilities provided a nominal solution to management issues.

The backlash against nurse-midwives has been powerful and punitive

(Sullivan and Weitz, 1988; Arnup, Levesque, and Pierson, 1990). Significant numbers have been forced entirely out of the practices for which they are trained and credentialed, primarily through increasing malpractice insurance rates and licensing regulations. This action has proven again the social and financial control of physicians within obstetrics/gynecology.

FUTURE DIRECTIONS

In the past, and in other countries today, men have often controlled the sexuality and reproduction of their "property" through physical as well as social and legal means: chastity belts (Davis, 1971), foot-binding (Daly, 1978), and clitoridectomy (still common today in many Moslem countries) (Hosken, 1976). In the United States today, forced sterilizations (CARASA, 1979), hysterectomies performed too frequently (Centers for Disease Control, 1980; Kjerulff et al., 1992), lack of Medicaid funding for abortion, and denial of access to lesbians for artificial insemination (Hornstein, 1984; Hubbard, 1990) are examples of the ways women's sexuality and reproduction are regulated. Not coincidentally, the medical establishment, particularly the decision-making portion dealing with women's reproduction, is strongly dominated by men.

Considering the history of male takeover of gynecology in the United States and current abuses, can it be expected that the new reproductive technologies, developed and controlled by a scientific and medical establishment dominated by men, will be completely positive for women? Technologies such as amniocentesis, chorionic villi biopsy, artificial insemination, and in vitro fertilization are heralded by the media as "liberating" women. They permit women who are older, who do not wish to have intercourse, or who have blocked oviducts to bear children. However, upon closer examination, each of these new technologies also has an oppressive side; each may also be used in a way to control or limit women's sexuality or reproductive access. Amniocentesis and chorionic villi biopsy may be used to abort a child of an unwanted sex, usually female (Roggencamp, 1984; Hoskins and Holmes, 1984; Hubbard, 1990). In most localities, artificial insemination is denied women who are unmarried or open about their lesbianism (Hornstein, 1984; Hubbard, 1990). In vitro fertilization is very expensive, $5,000 per insemination with a 23 percent chance of success, and often available only to married couples (Gold, 1985).

As with most technologies, intrinsically the new reproductive technologies are neither good nor bad; it is the way they are used that determines their potential for benefit or harm. The androcentric scientific and medical establishment creates and controls these technologies; one must evaluate them from a feminist perspective to begin to appreciate their full implications for women before their benefits or hazards can be assessed.

Amniocentesis, for example, has both its positive and negative aspects. Its benefits include the ability to detect some seventy abnormalities, including Trisomy 21, Edwards' Syndrome, and spina bifida (Ritchie, 1984), and peace of mind during the latter half of pregnancy based on the assumption that no genetic defects are present in the fetus, providing the test has been accurately administered, cultured, and read. Some of its risks include a 1.0–1.5 percent increased chance of miscarriage or fetal abnormalities, such as clubfoot or dislocated hip, breathing difficulties at birth, and Rh sensitization (Ritchie, 1984); necessity of a second-trimester abortion if the woman wishes to terminate the pregnancy after learning the results; the physical discomfort of the procedure; the psychological discomfort of waiting three to four weeks for the results; and the false sense of security arising from the assumption that most "defects" can be detected by the procedure when developmental and other nongenetic defects cannot be detected.

When amniocentesis is considered from the perspectives of class and religion, it is restricted mostly to middle-class women whose religious background has limited sanctions against abortion. The issue of amniocentesis raises questions about what it means to be labeled "abnormal" or defective in our society, and about who decides who is "normal," therefore worthy of life, and who is "abnormal," and should be aborted. Women of color have pointed out that other tests of normality (IQ) have often been used to screen out nonwhites and represent people of color as inferior (Chase, 1980).

This point becomes even clearer when international data are examined. In India (Chacko, 1982; Roggencamp, 1984) and China (Campbell, 1976), and probably in some clinics in the United States (Roggencamp, 1984; Hubbard, 1990), the results of amniocentesis are used as the basis for aborting female fetuses. All women react strongly to the fact that this reproductive technology may be used to define who is worthy of living, and that in many cases this decision would exclude women. Thus, the technology that has been represented by the media and medical profession as a benefit to women, that allows women to delay childbearing and still guarantee a healthy baby, may also be used to enforce societal restrictions on physical and mental norms and even limit women in subsequent generations.

Women have fought hard for their reproductive rights: choice of contraception, abortion, and sterilization. However, these procedures are still controlled by men, which means that they may also be used to manipulate women's sexuality.

The current use of surrogate mothers is a clear way in which women's bodies are used to produce the property of men (Ince, 1984). The new technologies that increase the chances of having a healthy baby place extreme pressure on the individual woman to produce a "perfect piece of property" (Hubbard, 1990). The information now available about the effects of alcohol, drugs, smoking, disease, and nutrition during pregnancy and the availability of amniocentesis and chorionic villi biopsy burden women with the guilt of bearing a child with a "defect." By placing the burden of guilt on individual women, men and society lose sight of their responsibility to care for these children. Although the vast majority of physical and mental disabilities are not due to diseases or abnormalities detectable by amniocentesis or to the maternal environment during pregnancy, the current trend leaves people with the impression that they are. Therefore, society as a whole feels that the woman is responsible for "producing" (or failing to abort) this "defective" child, and so must care for it (Hubbard, 1990). At the same time funding is reduced for nutritional needs and prenatal care for poor women, despite evidence demonstrating the role of poor nutrition and lack of care in producing defective children.

Obstetrics/gynecology is a specialty in which the male scientific and medical establishments have developed and used technologies for more than a century. Some of these technologies have greatly benefited women in their potential to save the lives of both mothers and babies. Once again, however, the difficulty is in their overuse by the medical profession to speed normal deliveries, make money, and enhance hospital procedure at the cost of a normal delivery by women who might not have needed medical intervention. The control of these technologies exemplifies the extent to which androcentrism permeates the only medical specialty currently devoted exclusively to women's health issues.

REFERENCES

Aeschylus. 1975. *The oresteia.* Trans. R. Fagles. New York: Viking Press.

Alexander, Nancy. 1993. Current and future status of contraception. Abstract published in *Journal of Women's Health* 2, no. 2:202.

Arditti, Rita; Duelli Klein, Renate; and Minden, Shelley. 1984. *Test-tube women: What future for motherhood?* London: Pandora Press.

Arms, Suzanne. 1977. *Immaculate deception: A new look at women and childbirth in America.* New York: Bantam Books.

Arnup, Katherine; Levesque, Andre; and Pierson, Ruth. 1990. *Delivering motherhood: Maternal ideologies and practices in the nineteenth and twentieth centuries.* New York: Routledge.

Association of American Medical Colleges. 1989. Addressing gender bias in interviews. *AAMC Women in Medicine Update* 3:3.

Banta, D., and Thacker, S. 1982. The risks and benefits of episiotomy: A review. *Birth* 9, no. 1:25–30.

Benokraitis, Nijole, and Feagin, Joe. 1986. *Modern sexism: Blatant, subtle and covert discrimination.* Englewood Cliffs, N.J.: Prentice Hall.

Biology and Gender Study Group. 1988. The importance of feminist critique for contemporary cell biology. In Nancy Tuana (ed.), *Feminism and science.* Bloomington and Indianapolis: Indiana University Press.

Boston Women's Health Book Collective. 1992. *The new our bodies, ourselves.* New York: Simon and Schuster.

Campbell, C. 1976. The manchild pill. *Psychology Today* (August):86–89.

CARASA (Committee for Abortion Rights and against Sterilization Abuse). 1979. *Women under attack: Abortion, sterilization and reproductive freedom.* New York: Author.

Carlson, Karen. 1991. Outcomes research on hysterectomy: The Maine Women's Health Study. *Women's Health Forum* 1, no. 1:1–2.

Centers for Disease Control. 1980. *Surgical sterilization surveillance: Hysterectomy in women aged 15–44, from 1970–1975.* Atlanta, Ga.: CDC.

Chacko, A. 1982. Too many daughters: India's drastic cure. *World Paper* (November):8–9.

Chalker, Rebecca, and Downer, Carol. 1992. *A woman's book of choices: Abortion, menstrual extraction, RU-486.* New York: Four Walls, Eight Windows Press.

Chase, A. 1980. *The legacy of Malthus.* Urbana: University of Illinois Press.

Corea, Gena, et al. (eds.). 1987. *Man-made women: How new reproductive technologies affect women.* Bloomington: Indiana University Press.

Corea, Gena, and Ince, S. 1978. Report of a survey of IVF clinics in the USA. In Patricia Spallone and Deborah L. Steinberg (eds.), *Made to order: The myth of reproductive and genetic progress.* Oxford: Pergamon Press.

Cowan, Belita. 1980. Ethical problems in government-funded contraceptive research. In Helen Holmes, Betty Hoskins, and Michael Gross (eds.), *Birth control and controlling birth: Women-centered perspectives,* pp. 37–46. Clifton, N.J.: Humana Press.

Daly, Mary. 1978. *Gyn/Ecology: The metaethics of radical feminism.* Boston: Beacon Press.

Darty, T., and Potter, S. 1984. Lesbians and contemporary health care systems: Oppression and opportunity. In T. Darty and S. Potter (eds.), *Women identified women.* Palo Alto, Calif.: Mayfield Publishing Company.

Davis, E. G. 1971. *The first sex.* New York: G. P. Putnam.

Direcks, Anita, and Hoen, Ellen. 1986. DES: The crime continues. In Kathleen McDonnell (ed.), *Adverse effects: Women and the pharmaceutical industry,* pp. 41–50. Toronto, Canada: The Women's Press.

Dreifus, Claudia. 1975. Sterilizing the poor. *The Progressive* (December):13.

———. 1978. *Seizing our bodies.* New York: Vintage Books.

Ehrenreich, Barbara, and English, Deirdre. 1978. *For her own good.* New York: Anchor Press.

Eicher, E. M., and Washburn, L. 1986. Genetic control of primary sex determination in mice. *Annual Review of Genetics* 20:327–360.

Fausto-Sterling, Anne. 1985; revised 1992. *Myths of gender: Biological theories about women and men.* New York: Basic Books.

Fee, Elizabeth. 1981. Is feminism a threat to scientific objectivity? *International Journal of Women's Studies:* 4:213–233.

———. 1982. A feminist critique of scientific objectivity. *Science for the People* 14, no. 4:8.

Gold, M. (1985). The baby makers. *Science, 85* 6, no. 3:26–38.

Goldzieher, Joseph W.; Moses, Louis; Averkin, Eugene; Scheel, Cora; and Taber, Ben. 1971a. A placebo-controlled double-blind crossover investigation of the side effects attributed to oral contraceptives. *Fertility and Sterility* 22, no. 9:609–623.

———. 1971b. Nervousness and depression attributed to oral contraceptives: A double-blind, placebo-controlled study. *American Journal of Obstetrics and Gynecology* 22:1013–1020.

Greenblatt, Ruth, and Schuman, Paula. 1993. Sexually transmitted diseases and AIDS in the 1990's: The women's epidemic. Abstract published in *Journal of Women's Health* 2, no. 2:204.

Guillemin, Jeanne. 1981. Babies by Caesarian: Who chooses, who controls? *The Hastings Center Report* 11, no. 3:15–18.

Hamilton, Jean. 1985. Avoiding methodological biases in gender-related research. In *Women's health report of the Public Health Service Task Force on Women's Health Issues.* Washington, D.C.: U.S. Department of Health and Human Service Public Service.

Haraway, Donna. 1978. Animal sociology and a natural economy of the body politic, Part I: A political physiology of dominance; and Animal sociology and a natural economy of the body politic, Part II: The past is the contested zone: Human nature and theories of production and reproduction in primate behavior studies. *Signs: Journal of Women in Culture and Society* 4, no. 1:21–60.

Harding, Sandra. 1986. *The science question in feminism.* Ithaca, N.Y.: Cornell University Press.

Harrison, Michelle. 1992. Con: Women's health as a specialty: A deceptive solution. *Journal of Women's Health* 1, no. 2:102–106.

Henderson, I. C., and Wender, R. C. 1991. Breast cancer. *American Cancer Society Newsletter* 2:1.

Herschberger, Ruth. 1970. *Adam's rib.* New York: Harper and Row. (Originally published 1948.)

Holmes, H. B. 1981. Reproductive technologies: The birth of women-centered analysis. In Helen B. Holmes et al. (eds.), *The custom-made child?* Clifton, N.J.: Humana Press.

Holmes, Helen B.; Hoskins, B. B.; and Gross, M. 1980. *Birth control and controlling birth: Women-centered perspectives.* Clifton, N.J.: Humana Press.

Hornstein, F. 1984. Children by donor insemination: A new choice for lesbians. In Rita Arditti, Renate Duelli Klein, and Shelley Minden (eds.), *Test-tube women,* pp. 373–381. London: Pandora Press.

Hosken, F. P. 1976. *WIN News* 2:3.

Hoskins, B., and Holmes, H. 1984. Technology and prenatal femicide. In Rita Arditti, Renate Duelli Klein, and Shelley Minden (eds.), *Test-tube women,* pp. 237–255. London: Pandora Press.

Hubbard, Ruth. 1990. *The politics of women's biology.* New Brunswick, N.J.: Rutgers University Press.

Ince, S. 1984. Inside the surrogate industry. In Rita Arditti, Renate Duelli Klein, and Shelley Minden (eds.), *Test-tube women,* pp. 99–116. London: Pandora Press.

Johnson, Karen. 1992. Pro: Women's health: Developing a new interdisciplinary specialty. *Journal of Women's Health* 2:101.

Jost, A. 1947. Recherches sur la differenciation sexuelle de l'embryon de Lapin. I. Introduction et embryologie genitale normale. *Archives d'Anatomie Microscopique et de Morphologie Experimentale* 36:151–200.

———. 1958. Embryonic sexual differentiation. In H. W. Jones and W. W. Scott (eds.), *Hermaphroditism, genital anomalies and related endocrine disorders.* Baltimore: Williams and Wilkins.

Keeton, W. C. 1976. *Biological science.* 3rd ed. New York: W. W. Norton.

Keller, Evelyn Fox. 1985. *Reflections on gender and science.* New Haven, Conn.: Yale University Press.

Kitzinger, Sheila. 1981. *Episiotomy: Physical and emotional aspects.* London: The National Childbirth Trust.

Kjerulff, K. H., et al. 1992. Hysterectomy: An examination of a common surgical procedure. *Journal of Women's Health* 1, no. 2:141–148.

Klein, Renate; Dumble, Lynette; and Raymond, Janice. 1992. *RU-486 misconceptions, myths, and morals.* Cambridge, Mass.: Institute on Women and Technology.

LaCheen, Cary. 1986. Population control and the pharmaceutical industry. In Kathleen McDonnell (ed.), *Adverse effects*, pp. 89–136. Toronto, Canada: Women's Press.

Lorber, Judith. 1988. *In vitro* fertilization and gender politics. In E. H. Baruch, A. S. D'Adams, Jr., and J. Seager (eds.), *Embryos, ethics, and women's rights*, pp. 117–133. New York: Haworth Press.

Marieskind, Helen. 1979. *An evaluation of Cesarean section in the United States.* Report of the Task Force, Cesarean Childbirth. Bethesda, Md.: NIH publication no. 82–2067, p. 25.

Martin, Emily. 1991. The egg and the sperm: How science has constructed a romance based on stereotypical male-female roles. *Signs* 16, no. 3:485–501.

Merchant, Carolyn. 1979. *The death of nature: Women, ecology and the scientific revolution.* New York: Harper and Row.

Minkoff, H.; Moreno, Jonathan; and Powderly, Kathleen. 1992. Fetal protection and women's access to clinical trials. *Journal of Women's Health* 1, no. 2:137–140.

Mintz, Morton. 1985. *At any cost: Corporate greed, women and the Dalkon Shield.* New York: Pantheon Books.

Muller, Charlotte. 1990. *Health care and gender.* New York: Russell Sage Foundation.

Murphy, J. 1984. Egg farming and women's future. In Rita Arditti, Renate Duelli Klein, and Shelley Minden (eds.), *Test-tube women*, pp. 68–75. London: Pandora Press.

Pappert, Ann. 1986. The rise and fall of the IUD. In Kathleen McDonnell (ed.), *Adverse effects*. Toronto, Canada: Women's Press.

Pokras, R. 1989. Hysterectomy: Past, present and future. *Statistical Bulletin* 70:12–21. New York: Metropolitan Life and Affiliated Companies.

Pokras, R., and Hufnagel, V. G. 1988. Hysterectomy in the United States, 1965–84. *American Journal of Public Health* 78, no. 7:852–853.

Postgate, J. 1973. Bat's chance in hell. *New Scientist* 5:11–16.

Rennie, Susan. 1993. Breast cancer prevention: Diet vs. drugs. *Ms.* 3, no. 6:38–46.

Ritchie, M. 1984. Taking the initiative: Information versus technology in pregnancy. In Rita Arditti, Renate Duelli Klein, and Shelley Minden (eds.), *Test-tube women*, pp. 402–413. London: Pandora Press.

Rodriguez-Trias, Helen. 1980. Sterilization abuse. In Rita Arditti, Pat Brennan, and Steve Cavrak (eds.), *Science and liberation*, pp. 113–117. Boston: South End Press.

Roggencamp, V. 1984. Abortion of a special kind: Male sex selection in India. In Rita Arditti, Renate Duelli Klein, and Shelley Minden (eds.), *Test-tube women*, pp. 266–278. London: Pandora Press.

Rothman, Barbara K. 1982. Awake and aware, or false consciousness: The cooptation of childbirth reforms in America. In S. Romalis (ed.), *Childbirth: Alternatives to medical control.* Austin: University of Texas Press.

Ruzek, Sheryl. 1978. *The women's health movement.* New York: Praeger.

Schatten, Gerald, and Schatten, Heide. 1983. The energetic egg. *The Sciences* 23, no. 5:28–34.

Seaman, Barbara, and Seaman, Gideon. 1977. *Women and the crisis in sex hormones.* New York: Bantam Books.

Selwyn, P. A., et al. 1989. Prospective study of human immunodeficiency virus infection and pregnancy outcomes in intravenous drug users. *Journal of the American Medical Association* 261:1289–1294.

Sullivan, Deborah, and Weitz, Rose. 1988. *Labor pains: Modern midwives and home birth.* New Haven, Conn.: Yale University Press.

Taylor, R. 1979. *Medicine out of control.* Melbourne: Sun Books.

Tuana, Nancy. 1988. The weaker seed: The sexist bias of reproductive theory. In Nancy Tuana (ed.), *Feminism and science.* Bloomington: Indiana University Press.

Vasquez-Calzada, José. 1973. La Esterilizacion Femenina en Puerto Rico. *Revista de Ciencias Sociales* 17, no. 3:281–308.

Veatch, Robert M. 1971. Experimental pregnancy. *Hastings Center Report* 1:2–3.

Wallis, Lila. 1992. Commentary: Women's health: A specialty? Pros and cons. *Journal of Women's Health* 2:107.

Wallis, Lila A. 1992. Women's health curriculum abstract for reframing women's health: Multidisciplinary Research and Practice Conference, October 15–17 workshop abstracts. Chicago: University of Illinois at Chicago Center for Research on Women and Gender.

Wertz, Richard, and Wertz, Dorothy. 1989. *Lying-in: A history of childbirth in America.* Revised ed. New Haven, Conn.: Yale University Press.

Wilson, Robert. 1966. *Feminine forever.* New York: M. Evans and Co.

Worcester, Nancy, and Whatley, Marianne. 1988. The response of the health care system to the women's health movement: The selling of women's health centers. In Sue V. Rosser (ed.), *Feminism in the science and health care professions.* Elmsford, N.Y.: Pergamon Press.

Wright, R. C. 1969. "Hysterectomy: Past, present and future." *Obstetrics and Gynecology* 33:560–563.

Zimmerman, B., et al. 1980. People's science. In Rita Arditti, Pat Brennan, and Steve Cavrak (eds.), *Science and liberation,* pp. 299–319. Boston: South End Press.

Part Two

IGNORING DIVERSITY AMONG WOMEN IN CLINICAL RESEARCH AND PRACTICE

CHAPTER FIVE

Elderly Women

Androcentrism permeates all phases of clinical research. This bias then becomes translated into diagnoses, treatments, and other medical practices that are less appropriate for women and ultimately for all people.

Elderly women, women of color, and lesbians experience the effects of sexism combined with racism, ageism, and/or homophobia. Not only does each group have needs that distinguish it from the other groups, but each also has different relationships and maintains different distances from the mainstream clinical research. Given the difficulties with androcentrism and the problems with making research on women's health a national priority, it is not surprising that research on the health of these diverse groups of women is virtually nonexistent.

For only one of these groups, elderly women, is there a recognized clinical specialty designated to address some of their health needs. Gerontology, a newly emerging field without a clear research agenda, has already demonstrated androcentrism by excluding women from its most comprehensive longitudinal study. However, it is easier to envision some of the problems of bias and exclusion from clinical research for elderly women since a specialty defining some of the issues for older people is available for critique.

The latest data from the Census Bureau underscore the dramatic increase in the elderly population in the United States: 12.5 percent of the population is sixty-five or older; the number of people over seventy-five is increasing more rapidly than any other segment of the population. Elderly women outnumber elderly men by a ratio of 2:1 (U.S. Bureau of the Census, 1991). Because women die later in life than men, they accumulate more acute, chronic diseases which tend to result in greater disability before death (Lewis, 1985) and greater out-of-pocket expenses than do the acute illnesses suffered more commonly by men (Sofaer and Abel, 1990). Their greater longevity also means that most women who serve as caretakers for a spouse when his health fails must rely on the support of health services, extended family, and friends during their own health care crises.

These data strongly suggest that elderly women will become an increasingly significant proportion of the population who will need a disproportionately large amount of health care. Research on diseases, maintenance of health and well-being, and successful, cost-efficient health care practices appropriate for elderly women should be accorded high priority on the national health care agenda. Ironically, the limited research in gerontology has tended to ignore women. For example, the Baltimore Longitudinal Study on Aging, the largest longitudinal study to assess the geriatric population, which was begun in 1958, included no women subjects for the first twenty years (Johnson, 1992). This omission delayed the discovery of the link among osteoporosis, calcium, estrogen, and progesterone.

As chapter 1 indicates, exclusion of women from clinical research and health agendas represents a long-standing problem in most specialties in medicine. Despite the fact that the geriatric population is overwhelmingly female, researchers in gerontology seem to ignore that fact when choosing topics for study and designing research protocols. In obstetrics/gynecology, the focus is on women of reproductive age. Elderly women are thus excluded from the research in the specialty devoted to women's health, as well as in gerontology.

Sexism and ageism combine and intertwine to push elderly women to the margins of clinical research. What are the effects of this marginalization on the choice of problems for study, approaches and methods, and the translation of theories and conclusions drawn from the data into practices for health care for elderly women?

CHOICE AND DEFINITION OF PROBLEMS FOR STUDY

In many ways, this section of this chapter could directly reiterate chapter 1, which explores the ways that androcentric bias affects the choice and definition of research problems for the health of women. The variable of age adds increased complexities to the bias in a variety of ways.

Hypotheses are not formulated to include the intersection of gender and age as a crucial part of the question being asked. As a rather dramatic example, four major studies exploring cardiovascular disease—the research on cholesterol-lowering drugs, the Multiple Risk Intervention Trial, the Health Professionals Follow-up Study, and the Physician's Health Study—included no women. Middle-aged men were used as the subjects because men develop heart disease at a younger age (ten to fifteen years earlier) than women. The subsequent interpretation of the research results was that women are not significantly affected by coronary heart disease.

In 1988, however, 380,000 women—almost as many women as men—died of coronary heart disease (National Center on Health Statistics, 1992). In assuming that this disease is not significant for women, researchers failed to take into account women's greater longevity. The conclusion that coronary heart disease does not strike men and women with equal frequency holds only when rates for middle-aged men are compared with rates for middle-aged women. When rates for men of all ages are compared with rates for women of all ages, the death rates are similar. A survey of the literature from 1961 to 1991 (Gurwitz, Nananda, and Avorn, 1992) revealed that women were included in only 18 percent of studies and the elderly in only 40 percent for medications to treat myocardial infarction.

Age-related variables such as decreasing levels of hormones may make "male" disease definitions for research on diseases that affect both men and women particularly invalid for elderly women. By age fifty-five, women are just as likely to have high blood pressure as men the same age. Almost twice as many women die from strokes as men. Women are 50 percent more likely than men to have dangerously high cholesterol levels. However, older women on low-fat diets do not experience the same decrease in low-density lipoprotein (LDL) cholesterol (bad cholesterol) and the same increase in high-density lipoprotein (HDL) cholesterol (good cholesterol) as older men on the same diets (Morgan, 1990). Presumably the decreasing levels of estrogen in postmenopausal woman eliminate the protection from strokes and other cardiovascular diseases found in the menstruating woman, but do not change the liver's metabolism of fats in women to make it similar to that of men. Since very little research has explored the relationship between hormone levels and liver function in postmenopausal females, the implications of this male-female difference are poorly understood (Morgan, 1990).

Diabetes and arthritis are two diseases which are problematic for both older men and women, but for which the changing hormone levels in women provide complications which have been studied insufficiently. Two decades ago, diabetes was more common in older women (Hamilton, 1985), but now that it has become more prevalent in older men, much research has been directed toward identifying the reasons for this increase. Although important, this research direction has left many of the interactions between diabetes and changing hormone levels in elderly women understudied. For example, it is known that diabetic women over forty are at higher risk for cystitis and for osteoporosis compared to nondiabetic older women and to younger diabetic women (Hamilton, 1985). Diabetic women also suffer increased symptoms of menopause which may be confused with insulin reaction symptoms. Profuse sweating, vaginal itching, and fatigue may all be due to an insulin reaction or to menopause (Porcino, 1983). The interaction between diabetes and estrogen level has not been well studied.

Unlike diabetes, arthritis is still more prevalent in the older female than the older male population. Despite suggestions from researchers (Yelin et al., 1984) that estrogen replacement might help to prevent or slow the progress of the disease, few studies have directly examined the levels of decreasing estrogen correlated with increasing arthritis symptoms.

Obstetrics/gynecology, the specialty devoted to women's reproductive health, has underfunded research on menopause and breast, uterine, and ovarian cancer. As discussed in the preceding chapter, obstetrics/gynecology has focused particularly on women of childbearing years and their health concerns revolving around heterosexual intercourse. By definition, elderly women are past the age of childbearing. Because of women's greater longevity and men's tendency to select women younger than themselves for sexual partners, many older women are not regularly engaging in heterosexual intercourse.

Perhaps the rapid increase in the rate of breast cancer, so that the lifetime risk for women is now one in nine (Johnson, 1993), can be partially explained by the fact that it is a disease of older women. The greatest risk factor for breast cancer appears to be age. The postmenopausal older woman is at higher risk because the longer a woman lives, the greater are her chances of developing this disease.

Similarly, the chances of contracting uterine cancer, including both endometrial and cervical cancer, increase with age. Regular Pap smears, effective in detection of cervical cancer, do not adequately detect endometrial cancer (Chambers, 1993). Tests such as the uterine biopsy or Milan Markley technique detect endometrial cancer more adequately, but they are painful, relatively expensive, and not given routinely. More research is needed on the reasons for the increase and methods to detect endometrial cancer in elderly women. Estrogen use in postmenopausal women correlates with increased risk of endometrial cancer (Hamilton, 1985; Henrich, 1993) and possibly breast cancer, although a recent review article (Henrich, 1992) refutes this. Although not the traditional focus of obstetrics/gynecology, research on the causes and detection of and treatment for endometrial cancer should become a higher priority because of the increased prescription of estrogens in postmenopausal women for osteoporosis.

Many studies (Ettinger el al., 1992; Budoff, 1980; Ford, 1986) suggest that progestins administered together with estrogens considerably reduce the risk of endometrial cancer. These same studies and others reveal that this same combination of hormones diminishes the effectiveness of estrogen in preventing atherosclerosis (Stampfer et. al., 1991) and may decrease its effectiveness in preventing osteoporosis (Ettinger et al., 1992). Effective dosage regimens for hormone replacement therapy as well as the effectiveness of diet, exercise, calcium supplements, smoking behaviors, and other lifestyle factors in preventing osteoporosis must be researched (Moore, Bonnick, and Roberts, 1993). Girls, adolescent women, and postmenopausal women must be included in the studies along with women of reproductive age to elucidate which factors at varying stages of the life cycle may contribute to the development of osteoporosis in elderly women.

Stereotypes about behaviors appropriate for or common among elderly women have led to inadequate study of significant health problems frequent in this group. The contribution of gender bias and appropriate behaviors to the underdiagnosis of alcoholism in women was examined in chapter 3. Although alcoholism and drug dependence in the elderly population have received little study (Hamilton, 1985), for elderly women the problem of age further complicates recognition of these problems. For most people in our society, including health care professionals, the image of a kindly old grandmother is incompatible with the image of an alcoholic or drug addict. This stereotyping leads not only to underdiagnosis but also to failure to study substance abuse problems in elderly women. Newer studies on alcohol use in the elderly (National Institute on Alcohol Abuse and Alcoholism, 1984) devote little or no attention to the elderly woman. Decreasing tolerance for alcohol and drugs with the changing metabolism due to aging, effect of lowered hormone levels on alcohol and drug blood levels and metabolism by the liver, and interactions with other, prescription drugs commonly taken by elderly women are among the baseline research information needed about the postmenopausal female population.

Stereotyped ideas which link sexuality in women with procreation and youth in our society have led many health care practitioners and researchers to assume that the elderly, and particularly elderly women, are not sexually active, do not wish to become so, and should not be, even if they wish to be. These misconceptions have led to living situations in nursing homes and with relatives without the possibility for the privacy needed to pursue sexual relationships. Fear of the aging process and little knowledge of the actual sexual activities and desires of elderly women represent further barriers to research (Butler and Butler, 1976). Some research has explored the causes of the more frequent vaginal, urethral, and bladder infections due to the less acidic vaginal secretions and atrophied vaginal walls that result from the loss of estrogen (National Institute on Aging, 1981; Butler and Butler, 1976). These may be problematic for postmenopausal women engaging in heterosexual intercourse. Although HRT may be a partial answer, little research has explored the effect of diet, exercise, vitamins, and actual sexual desire in alleviating these symptoms.

A different but equally pervasive stereotype may be responsible for the dearth of research on the nutritional needs of postmenopausal women. The link between women and food is strong in our culture. Women are associated with physically nurturing young children through lactation and with buying, cooking, and serving food to others. Perhaps the expectation that women will provide for the nutritional needs of the family coupled with the lack of importance that medicine has traditionally assigned to the role of proper nutrition in promoting health and preventing disease may explain the paucity of research on nutrition in older women. Baseline data have not been collected on such things as nutritional guidelines for women over sixty-five, the Minimum Daily Requirements (MDRs) of vitamins for women over sixty-five, and specialized diets to supplement nutrient deficiencies exacerbated by or caused by medications commonly given for chronic disorders experienced by many older women.

Research on nutritional contributions to and prevention of osteoporosis, cardiovascular disease, loss of lean body mass, and loss of immune system function remains minimal.

Factors experienced by elderly women and their families as significant for easing daily life and independent living have not been a major focus of research. Incontinence is the tenth leading cause of hospitalization for kidney and urologic diseases for women of all ages (Fourcroy and Weaver, 1993). It is also the second most common reason (dementia is first) that women are institutionalized in long-term care facilities; many families list incontinence as the pivotal factor for institutionalization, because of the difficulty in managing the condition at home (Ouslander et al., 1982). Although research on incontinence, its causes, and treatment is pursued, the priority accorded and funds allocated for the research do not reflect the extent of the problem for elderly women and their families.

Little research has examined causes of accidents, including accidental falls, to determine to what extent these are preventable. A 1979 study (not divided by gender) revealed that 7 percent of deaths from falls occurred in persons older than sixty-five; in persons over seventy-five, the percentage jumps sixfold (Rubenstein and Robbins, 1984). Hip fractures have an estimated mortality rate of 20–30 percent and result in chronic disability, since 13 percent of survivors never return to independent ambulation (Hersey et al., 1984). Research has not yet been able to elucidate whether falls cause hip fractures or vice versa. Since hip fractures occur primarily in women, with white females having twice the risk of other groups at every age (Hamilton, 1985), one wonders whether sexism and ageism have not blinded investigators to the importance of this research for the lives of elderly women and their families.

Approaches and Methods

The exclusion of elderly women as experimental subjects from research protocols definitely reflects ageism and sexism. Fear of teratogenic effects that might produce a deformed offspring and interference of fluctuating menstrual hormones provided the traditional rationale for exempting women from clinical drug trials and other male-only protocols. Once they pass menopause, however, elderly women no longer fit these descriptors; ageism thus becomes the sole rationale for their exclusion.

As stated earlier, elderly women outnumber elderly men by a ratio of approximately 2:1. While in younger age groups women hold the statistical status of a bare majority, they literally *are* the geriatric population. Given these statistical realities, it is difficult to ascribe the exclusion of women from gerontological studies to anything other than sexism.

Diversity of chronic disease states, as well as factors such as race, class, and sexual orientation, should also be considered in the selection of sample populations of women for gerontological studies. Bias in data that results from the failure to include women of diverse races, classes, and sexual orientations in studies of diseases in which one or more of those factors may be relevant to the risk frequency, manifestation, or progress of the disease has been discussed in other chapters of this volume.

Older women differ from their younger cohorts in the prevalence of certain diseases. The major health characteristics of women sixty-five and older include the greater prevalence of multiple long-term chronic illnesses that cause limitations in lifestyle (National Center on Health Statistics, 1982; Sofaer and Abel, 1990). Noninstitutionalized older women have a higher prevalence than adult women aged seventeen to sixty-four of visual and hearing impairments, hypertension, coronary heart disease, cerebrovascular disease, diabetes, impairments of the lower extremities and hip, chronic bronchitis, all diseases of the urinary system, anemia, and upper gastrointestinal disorders.

Although women live longer than men, older women die from the same major causes (heart disease, cancer, cardiovascular diseases, and accidents) as older men do (Hamilton, 1985). The greater longevity of older women means that often they suffer more than one of these chronic conditions for a lengthy period of time.

Failure to consider the diversity and multiplicity of chronic diseases in random samples of women used in a gerontological study may introduce various biases into the research. Many of these diseases lead to other secondary conditions which may confound research results if they are not considered when designing the experiment. For example, diabetes has multiple common secondary effects, particularly on the cardiovascular system, which indirectly affects the kidneys, eyes, and extremities. Including women with even mild cases of diabetes in the clinical testing of a drug to evaluate its effectiveness in treating cystitis would be likely to result in underrating the effectiveness of the drug. Since bladder infections are frequent and chronic in elderly diabetic women, indiscriminate and unintentional inclusion of such women in the research protocol with nondiabetic women may bias the results.

Interdisciplinary approaches combining methods from the behavioral, natural, and health sciences are essential for research on elderly women. Women's greater longevity means not only that they often suffer more chronic diseases than men, but also that often they must cope with them without the aid of a spouse or caretaker (Stone, Cafferata, and Sangl, 1986). Social factors such as living alone, fear of falling, and inability to shop for and cook nutritious foods may directly affect the progress of certain diseases in ways that rarely occur in a younger population.

Osteoporosis represents a critical health care issue for older women, for which methods from the health, behavioral, and natural sciences can contribute beneficial research approaches. Osteoporosis is the principal underlying cause of bone fractures, particularly in the spine, wrist, and hip, in postmenopausal women (Hamilton, 1985). One of the top seven diseases affecting older Americans, it is responsible for 1.3 million fractures per year (Moore, Bonnick, and Roberts, 1993). Because of the adverse conditions—ranging from back pain and vertebral compression to hospitalization, depression, and death from hip fractures—that may result from osteoporosis (Moore, Bonnick, and Roberts, 1993; National Institutes of Health, 1984), the threat of fractures promotes fears of loss of independence, additional falls, pain from further fractures, and hospitalization in older women and is estimated to add $10 billion annually to U.S. health care costs (Moore, Bonnick, and Roberts, 1993).

Since osteoporosis increases an older woman's chances of debilitating injury and the possibility for institutionalization and death (20 percent of patients with hip fractures die within the first year; only 30–35 percent recover complete independence after the first year [Cummings et al., 1984]), research into its prevention and treatment is crucial. Weight-bearing exercise, appropriate levels of calcium in the diet, and estrogen replacement (Seeman and Riggs, 1981; Ross et al., 1991) have all been implicated in preventing bone loss. Well-designed studies using approaches from the health, behavioral, and natural sciences must be undertaken to ascertain the effectiveness of each factor at different stages of the life cycle in preventing or halting the progress of the disease. Interdisciplinary approaches will also be useful in exploring the synergistic interactions among exercise, calcium, and estrogen in halting osteoporosis. NIH has recently announced a multidisciplinary, multi-institute intervention study, the Women's Health Initiative (Pinn and La Rosa, 1992), to address the major causes of death, disability, and frailty among middle-aged and older women. Cardiovascular disease, cancer, and osteoporosis are its major targets. In using all nine institutes and centers within the NIH as well as scientists, clinicians, and health care providers throughout the country, the study acknowledges the necessity for interdisciplinary approaches in this area.

THEORIES AND THEIR APPLICATIONS IN PRACTICE

The ageism and sexism which have led to bias in the choice and definition of research problems and in methodological approaches to study those problems become translated into medical practices based on the theories and conclusions drawn from the data. These practices may directly affect the accuracy of diagnosis and immediate application of surgical procedures and technologies which may make a difference between life and death for some elderly women.

Excessive focus on male research subjects and definition of some diseases as "male" diseases has led to the underdiagnosis and treatment of these diseases in elderly women. In a 1991 study in Massachusetts and Maryland, Ayanian and Epstein (1991) demonstrated that women were significantly less likely than men to undergo coronary angioplasty, angiography, or surgery when admitted to the hospital with a diagnosis of myocardial infarction, unstable or stable angina, chronic ischemic heart disease, or chest pain. This significant difference remained even when variables such as race, age, economic status, and other chronic diseases such as diabetes and heart failure were controlled for. A similar study (Steingart et al., 1991) revealed that women had angina before myocardial infarction as frequently as and with more debilitating effects than men, yet women are referred for cardiac catheterization only half as often. These and other similar studies led Bernadine Healy, a cardiologist and director of the National Institutes of Health, to characterize the diagnosis of coronary heart disease in women as the Yentl syndrome: "Once a woman showed that she was just like a man, by having coronary artery disease or a myocardial infarction, then she was treated as a man should be" (Healy, 1991, p. 274). Since myocardial infarction is the leading cause of death among women in the United States (Healy, 1991), and since it is equally frequent in older men and women, the failure to recognize and treat it adequately leads to unnecessary deaths in some elderly women. Similar problems in recognition and treatment of alcoholism, nutritional deficiency, and sexual dysfunction in elderly women occur because society or the medical profession perceives these as diseases of men, as incompatible with female social roles, or as incompatible with women of particular races or classes.

Focus on male research subjects and definition of some diseases as "male" diseases has also led to the development of surgical procedures and technologies that are inappropriate for elderly women. Studies revealed that a much higher percentage of women than men died after coronary bypass surgery (Douglas and Brest, 1989; Golding and Groves, 1976). Certainly the slower response of the medical profession in providing appropriate procedures for women presenting with myocardial infarction (Douglas and Brest, 1989; Murdaugh and O'Rourke, 1988; Greenland et al., 1991) and other heart disease suggests that women undergoing coronary bypass surgery may have more chronic, untreated heart disease than the men who undergo the surgery (Ayanian and Epstein, 1991; Steingart et al., 1991). The relatively more advanced average age of women compared to men (Robinson et al., 1988) undergoing the surgery may also be a factor contributing to their higher death rate, although women's greater longevity may partially attenuate the importance of age. The 1976 study by Golding and Groves revealed that a major factor was surgeons' inexperience in performing the operation on the smaller hearts, with smaller veins, and in the more confined pericardial cavities of women's bodies as compared to men's bodies. Because the research on bypassing blocked coronary arteries was conceived to study a problem of significance for men and undertaken using men as experimental subjects, the techniques and skill of the surgeons were honed for the body of a middle-aged man. A particular irony resulting from this initial bias is that many surgeons are reluctant to try the operation on women now that surgical skill (based on practice) is known to be a contributing factor to the higher death rates in women. The study (Kelsey et al., 1993) demonstrating a death rate from angioplasty ten times higher for women than for men is likely to result in fewer angioplasties performed in women. Exclusion of women as subjects at earlier stages when techniques are being developed and perfected may preclude the real effectiveness of these treatments for women ever being known.

Similar problems may arise with medications. Not only are most medications tested on men, but the dosages are calibrated using the body weight and metabolism of young and middle-aged men. Little research has examined the effectiveness of various medications in women, particularly the dosages for elderly women, who have different metabolic rates, weights, and hormone levels than younger women. The 1992 study (Gurwitz, Nananda, and Avorn, 1992) published in the *Journal of the American Medical Association* which documented the exclusion of women from 82 percent of medication trials to treat myocardial infarction and the exclusion of the elderly from 60 percent of such trials concluded that their omission meant that the effectiveness of medication was unknown for those groups most vulnerable to myocardial infarction. Perhaps the ineffectiveness in treating diseases or extreme side effects of some drugs encountered by elderly women may be the result of inappropriate dosage levels rather than improper kind of medication.

A holistic view of the elderly woman, including her social, economic, and living situation, must be considered when translating research into health care practice. Because of increased longevity and marriage patterns whereby women traditionally marry men who are older than they are, many elderly women live alone; substantial numbers of women face social isolation and economic problems. Treatments for disease and promotion of health which fail to take into account these factors that result from gender and age are less likely to be successful for elderly women (Jecker, 1991; Lutz, 1989; Clancy and Massion, 1992). For example, a male cardiac patient who has a wife to supervise his medications, run errands, help him in dressing, bathing, and going to the bathroom, while also taking care of the house and cooking, can be released from the hospital much earlier than a female cardiac patient who lives alone. Constrained economic circumstances may preclude her from hiring private nursing care and individuals to help with household chores. Her own relative immobility from osteoporosis or partial deafness may have restricted her to relative social isolation. This restriction coupled with the multiple chronic illnesses suffered by her contemporaries means that none of her friends may be able to assume the task of caretaker or even run an occasional errand for her.

The relatively high death rates of elderly women compared to elderly men after hospitalization, not only for cardiac problems (Low, 1993) but also for hip fractures, may be attributable largely to social factors. Absence of caretakers may result in women trying to cope alone or being institutionalized when they could live at home with help. Either result may lead to earlier death for the elderly woman (Boogaard and Briody, 1985; Conn, Taylor, and Abele, 1991; Sharpe, Clark, and Janz, 1991).

Sexism and ageism have biased the choice of problems for study, experimental approaches, and theories as translated into health care practice to push elderly women to the margins of the national health research agenda. This peripheralization represents more than an academic problem of research bias. It represents a cost—a cost to the American taxpayers for increased institutionalization in nursing homes and hospital care, and a cost to elderly women in terms of increased suffering and death.

REFERENCES

Ayanian, J. A., and Epstein, A. M. 1991. Differences in the use of procedures between women and men hospitalized for coronary heart disease. *New England Journal of Medicine* 325:221–225.

Boogaard, M. A. K., and Briody, M. E. 1985. Comparison of the rehabilitation of men and women post-myocardial infarction. *Journal of Cardiopulmonary Rehabilitation* 5:379–384.

Budoff, Penny. 1980. *No more menstrual cramps and other good news.* New York: Putnam and Sons.

Butler, R. N., and Butler, M. I. 1976. *Love and sex after sixty.* New York: Harper and Row.

Chambers, Setsuko. 1993. Abnormal Pap smear and bleeding in the reproductive age woman. Abstract published in *Journal of Women's Health* 2, no. 2:203.

Clancy, Carolyn, and Massion, Charlea. 1992. American women's health care: A patchwork quilt with gaps. *Journal of the American Medical Association* 268, no. 14:1918–1920.

Conn, V. S.; Taylor, S. G.; and Abele, P. B. 1991. Myocardial infarction survivors: Age and gender differences in physical health, psychosocial state and regimen adherence. *Journal of Advanced Nursing* 16:1026–1034.

Cummings, S. R.; Kelsey, J. L.; Nevitt, M. C.; et al. 1985. Epidemiology of osteoporosis and osteoporotic fractures. *Epidemiology Review* 7:178–208.

Douglas, P. S., and Brest, A. N. 1989. *Heart disease in women.* Philadelphia: F. A. Davis Co.

Ettinger, Bruce, et al. 1992. Low-dosage micronized 17B-estradiol prevents bone loss in postmenstrual women. *American Journal of Obstetrics and Gynecology* 166, no. 2 (February):479–488.

Ford, Anne Rochon. 1986. Hormones: Getting out of hand. In Kathleen McDonnell (ed.), *Adverse effects: Women and the pharmaceutical industry,* pp. 27–40. Toronto, Ontario: The Women's Press.

Fourcroy, Jean L., and Weaver, Dona J. 1993. Female urologic disorders. Abstract published in the *Journal of Women's Health* 2, no. 2:202.

Golding, L. R., and Groves, L. K. 1976. Results of coronary artery surgery in women. *Cleveland Clinical Quarterly* 43:113–115.

Greenland, P.; Reicher-Reiss, H.; Goldbourt, U.; and Behar, S. (Israeli SPRINT investigators). (1991). In-hospital and 1-year mortality in 1,524 women after myocardial infarction. *Circulation* 83:484–491.

Gurwitz, Jerry H.; Nananda, F. Colonel; and Avorn, Jerry. 1992. The exclusion of the elderly and women from clinical trials in acute myocardial infarction. *Journal of the American Medical Association* 268, no. 11:1407–1422.

Hamilton, Jean. 1985. Guidelines for avoiding methodological and policy-making biases in gender-related health research. *Women's health: Report of the Public Health Service Task Force on Women's Health Issues* 2:IV-54–IV-64.

Healy, Bernadine. 1991. The Yentl syndrome. *New England Journal of Medicine* 325:274–276.

Henrich, Janet. 1992. The postmenopausal estrogen/breast cancer controversy. *Journal of the American Medical Association* 268, no. 14:1900–1902.

Henrich, Janet B. 1993. Health issues in menopausal women. Abstract from the First Annual Congress on Women's Health. *Journal of Women's Health* 2, no. 2:207.

Hersey, J. C., et al. 1984. Aging and health promotion: Marketing research for public education (282–83–0105). SRA Technologies and Porter, Novelli and Associates for the Office of Disease Prevention and Health Promotion, the National Institute on Aging and the National Cancer Institute, May, (a) pp. I-41–I-48.

Jecker, N. S. 1991. Age-based rationing and women. *Journal of the American Medical Association* 266:3012–3015.

Johnson, Karen. 1992. Pro: Women's health: Developing a new interdisciplinary specialty. *Journal of Women's Health* 1, no. 2:95–100.

Johnson, Tracy. 1993. A women's health research agenda. *Journal of Women's Health* 2, no. 2:95–98.

Kelsey, Sheryl, et al. 1993. Results of percutaneous transluminal coronary angioplasty in women: 1985–86 National Heart, Lung, and Blood Institutes Coronary Angioplasty Registry. *Circulation* 87, no. 3:720–727.

Lewis, M. 1985. Older women and health: An overview. *Women and Health* 10, nos. 2/3:1–16.

Low, Kathryn G. 1993. Recovery from myocardial infarction and coronary artery bypass surgery in women: Psychosocial factors. *Journal of Women's Health* 2, no. 2:133–139.

Lutz, M. E. 1989. Women, work and preventive health care: An exploratory study of the efficacy of HMO membership. *Women Health* 15:21–33.

Moore, Donnica; Bonnick, S. L.; and Roberts, M. 1993. Osteoporosis: A women's health priority. Abstract published in *Journal of Women's Health* 2, no. 2:207.

Murdaugh, C. L., and O'Rourke, R. A. 1988. Coronary heart disease in women: Special considerations. *Current Problems in Cardiology* 13:45–142.

National Center for Health Statistics. 1982. Use of health services by women 65 years of age and older. Series 13, No. 59, (a) pp. 1–7.

National Center on Health Statistics. 1992. *Health United States, 1991.* Hyattsville, Md.: U.S. Public Health Service.

National Institute on Aging. 1981. Sexuality in later life. Bethesda, Md.: Age Page.

National Institute on Alcohol Abuse and Alcoholism. 1984. Alcohol and the elderly (special issue [October]). Alcohol World 8:(ADM)84–151, pp. 1–64, Rockville, Md.

National Institutes of Health. 1984. NIH consensus development draft conference statement: Osteoporosis, pp. 8–9. Bethesda, Md.

Ouslander, J., et al. 1982. Urinary incontinence in elderly nursing home patients. *Journal of the American Medical Association* 248 (September):1194–1198.

Pinn, Vivian, and LaRosa, Judith. 1992. *Overview: Office of Research on Women's Health.* Bethesda, Md.: National Institutes of Health.

Porcino, J. 1983. *Growing older, getting better.* Reading, Pa.: Addison-Wesley Publishing Company.

Robinson, K.; Conroy, R. M.; Mulcah, R.; and Hickey, N. 1988. Risk factors and in-hospital course of first episode myocardial infarction or acute coronary insufficiency in women. *Journal of the American College of Cardiologists* 11:932–936.

Ross, P. D.; Davis, J. W.; Epstein, R. S.; and Wasnigh, R. D. 1991. Pre-existing fracture and bone mass predict vetebral fracture incidence in women. *Annals of Internal Medicine* 114:919–923.

Rubenstein, L., and Robbins, A. 1984. Falls in the elderly: A clinical perspective. *Geriatrics* 39:67–78.

Seeman, E., and Riggs, B. L. 1981. Dietary prevention of bone loss in the elderly. *Geriatrics* 36:71–79.

Sharpe, P. A.; Clark, N. M.; and Janz, N. K. 1991. Differences in the impact and management of heart disease between older men and women. *Women Health* 17:25–43.

Sofaer, S., and Abel, E. 1990. Older women's health and financial vulnerability: Implications of the Medicare benefit structure. *Women Health* 16:47–67.

Stampfer, M. J.; Colditz, G. A.; Willett, W. D.; et al. 1991. Postmenopausal estrogen therapy and cardiovascular disease. *New England Journal of Medicine* 325:756–762.

Steingart, R. M.; Packer, M.; Hamm, P.; et al. 1991. Sex differences in the management of coronary artery disease. *New England Journal of Medicine* 325:226–230.

Stone, R.; Cafferata, G. L.; and Sangl, J. 1986. *Caregivers of the frail elderly: A national profile.* Rockville, Md.: National Center for Health Services Research.

U.S. Bureau of the Census. 1991. *Statistical abstract of the United States: 1991.* 111th ed. Washington, D.C.: Government Printing Office.

Yelin, E., et al. 1984. Arthritis policy and the elderly. San Francisco: University of California, Aging Health Policy Center.

CHAPTER SIX

Women of Color

Racism intertwines with sexism and economics to move health care issues for women of color to the far margins, or to move them entirely out of the national agenda for clinical research. Their gender and their color doubly remove them from the white male, from whose perspective the research agenda is formulated and whose body serves as the norm from which deviations are calculated. When included, women of color too often become misused as subjects in experiments which either lend credence to racial stereotypes or fail to distinguish true health problems among races.

Many of the health and disease concerns of women of color overlap with those of white women. As the preceding chapters in this volume demonstrate, health concerns of white women have only recently begun to be a focus of the national research agenda. It was only in September 1990 that the Office of Research on Women's Health was established, and in late 1991 that the first permanent director of that office was hired.

Women of color also face many of the same problems with health and disease as do the men of their racial and ethnic groups. Men of color have not shared the central spotlight for research with white men. The first Office for Minority Health Affairs was not established until 1991.

The recent dates for the establishment of these two offices indicate the tardiness of the federal government in officially recognizing that the majority of its population, who are men of color and women, must be included in research along with white men. On March 9, 1994, the NIH published guidelines in the Federal Register on the inclusion of women and minorities in research involving human subjects. Women of color are in a unique position: their race connects them with the Office of Minority Affairs, and their gender connects them with the Office of Research on Women's Health. Perhaps this double focus will bring minority women's health concerns to the forefront of the agenda for the first time. It would be tragic if instead women of color became the focus of neither office, permitting their health concerns to again slip through the cracks of the research agenda.

Racism and sexism have combined to severely limit advances in health care for women of color. The dearth of research in general and the often delimitative nature of this research have yielded only meager, and in many cases unreliable, data regarding frequency and cause of diseases, exacerbation of illness by environmental factors, and effective treatments for promoting health and preventing disease in women of color. Some complications of racism and sexism have effectively invalidated such research in the past. A major problem has been that the phrase "women of color" is too often taken to mean a coherent group when in fact it includes women of extremely diverse racial and ethnic backgrounds who are not closely related to each other genetically or culturally. They may, therefore, differ more from each other than they do from white women. The concept of race as used by the Census Bureau and as based on self-classification by respondents (African-American, Asian-American, American Indian and Alaska Native, and Hispanic) sets up a false dichotomy: white women/women of color.

Considerable diversity also may exist within each group. For example, Asians and Pacific Islanders in the United States include more than twenty-five subgroups, such as Chinese, Filipinos, Japanese, Indians, Koreans, Vietnamese, Hawaiians, Samoans, Guamanians, Burmese, Cambodians, Laotians, Thais, and others (Manley et al., 1985). Although they share an origin in Asia and the Pacific Islands, they have different cultures, languages, and probably gene pools. Since the majority of Asians and Pacific Islanders in the United States today are first-generation immigrants, virtually no baseline data exist on the health of these women. Less explicable is the fact that even for those whose ancestors immigrated to this country more than a century ago, only limited baseline data exist.

The Hispanic population also does not represent a homogeneous ethnic group. Mexican-Americans, Puerto Ricans, Cubans, and individuals from sixteen other Latin American countries and Spain speak Spanish but have their origins in very different cultures and countries. Since many Chicanas and those from other Latin American cultures are also first-generation Americans, there is little history of research and few baseline data for Hispanic women either.

For American Indian and Alaska Native women, the first female Americans, predating not only white women but also white men, short tenure in the United States cannot be used to explain the absence of research (and their poor health). Similarly, the African-American population, originally transported to the United States against its will, is the oldest and most stable nonindigenous minority group. Yet little good research has explored Black women's health, despite the fact that, in many ways, Black women are the most vulnerable of all minority women (Manley et al., 1985).

In the rare cases where women of color have been the focus of clinical research, at best the results have yielded little or inadequate information about health and disease processes. At worst the women have served as guinea pigs for clinical trials of unsafe drugs or for experiments to document possible biological bases for social ills.

Many studies (White, 1990; Manley et al., 1985; Braithwaite and Taylor, 1992; Avery, 1992) have defined access to health care as the controlling factor for health and disease in the lives of minority women. Researchers have also produced a considerable body of work that examines the relationship among poverty, access, and health care for minority women (Alcena, 1992; Braithwaite and Taylor, 1992). The median survival rate for white females is 78.9 years and for Black females 73.0 years (Alcena, 1992).

Most diseases, such as hypertension, cardiovascular disease, alcoholism, certain cancers, and diabetes, as well as the increased rates of homicide and maternal and infant mortality responsible for the shortened life span of women of color compared to white women, may largely be the result of poverty and inadequate access to health care. However, individuals contract these diseases as a result of interactions between genetic and "lifestyle" factors, including environmental risks such as poverty. Virtually no research has attempted through controlled, clinical trials to determine the extent to which genetic factors compared to "lifestyle" factors usually related to class such as diet, smoking, exercise, living near toxic or polluted sites, and medications contribute to decreased longevity for women of color. For example, the increasing cancer rates among Black women (Boston Women's Health Book Collective, 1992; Avery, 1992) are now frequently attributed to the stress that people of color, particularly women (Adisa, 1990; Alcena, 1992), experience in our society. Although women of color apparently do bear increased stress which probably does contribute to their increasing cancer rates, there does not seem to have been a well-controlled study that examines the various factors necessary for drawing such a conclusion. The complex, interlocking factors of race, gender, and class, along with other factors such as family history of cancer and number of stressful "lifestyle" factors (death of spouse, divorce, moving, substance abuse, being lesbian), would have to be compared between women of the same class, with similar family histories of cancer and a similar "stress burden" but of different races, for the claim to be validated.

Failure to disentangle the complex, interlocking variables of race, class, and gender, as well as other factors relevant to the health or disease issue under study, introduces bias into the experiment. Since these factors are often highly correlated and since the sample populations of women of color are relatively small, much clinical research has been flawed by the failure to account for these factors. Such flaws may bias the choice and definition of problems for study, experimental approaches used, and theories and conclusions drawn from the data in clinical research on health and disease in women of color.

Choice and Definition of Problems for Study

Women of color have not been accorded a major priority in the national health agenda. Their absence or exclusion is manifested in the choice and definition of problems selected for research in a variety of ways. And when women of color *are* included, the choice and definition of problems must be more fully examined.

Race and gender are not given conscious consideration when experimental subjects are selected for inclusion in research projects. When women are excluded from experiments, as some studies have indicated that they may be as much as 80 percent of the time (Gurwitz, Nananda, and Avorn, 1992), women of color are also excluded. As discussed particularly in chapters 1 and 5, this exclusion leads the entire population to have misperceptions and inadequate information about life-threatening conditions which are of particular concern to women of color such as myocardial infarction and AIDS.

In other cases, women of color are excluded from experiments in which Caucasian women serve as the female subjects (Minkoff, Moreno, and Powderly, 1992). If it is not stated in the experimental protocol that only white females were used and if the data are then extrapolated to all females, this may be inappropriate for diseases or conditions that have different frequencies and manifestations in different racial and ethnic groups.

Lumping together women from different racial/ethnic groups as experimental subjects without including them in representative sample sizes proportional to their numbers in the overall population may bias results regarding frequency of certain diseases in the population. For example, testing a sample of mammograms from a group composed of 50 percent white women and 50 percent Black women of age fifty-five to estimate the frequency of breast cancer in the U.S. population would probably result in an underestimate of the frequency in the total female population because Black women exhibit a lower incidence of breast cancer than white women. Consequently, cost projections to fund early treatment programs for breast cancer which used this frequency would underestimate the number of women needing such treatment because Black women constitute 12 percent rather than 50 percent of the female population. Similarly, about 90 percent of lupus patients are women (Shulman, 1985). Using a population sample consisting of 50 percent white women and 50 percent Black women to test strategies effective in treatment of systemic lupus erythematosus would also prove inaccurate, since lupus appears to be three times more common in Black women than white women (Manley et al., 1985; Jones, 1990). Some data from outside the mainland United States (Shulman, 1985; Pike, 1993) suggest that lupus may be unusually common in Chinese women. Failure to include or exclude women with Chinese ancestry might also bias the test.

Lumping together women from different racial and ethnic backgrounds without considering the frequency of certain genes in racial/ethnic groups that may enhance or inhibit certain disease conditions may also introduce bias into the results. Take, for example, a longitudinal experiment attempting to measure the effectiveness in preventing osteoporosis of drinking milk compared to taking calcium tablets. Assume that since the experimenters know of data suggesting that Black and American Indian women have lower rates of osteoporosis, they include only Caucasian and Asian women in their study. Failure to recognize that the high rate of glucose-6-phosphate dehydrogenase deficiency in the Asian population is likely to mean that a substantial proportion of the Asian women in the group drinking milk will not be able to tolerate it, and thus will lose the benefit from the calcium in the milk, may introduce a flaw. Lack of knowledge of the relatively high frequency of this genetic difference in the Asian population may bias the experiment toward calcium pills.

Simply including women without regard for their racial and ethnic background or consciousness of genetic differences in those groups as experimental subjects may bias the data collection. Explicit attention to including women in sample sizes representative of their numbers in ethnic/racial groups in the overall population will lead to more accurate experimental designs which will yield reliable data.

Women's health priorities for research have been defined using the white female as the norm. Just as the overall national health priorities suffer from using the white male and his diseases as the norm, the emerging national priorities for women's health reflect the priorities of the white female.

Dr. Bernadine Healy, director of the National Institutes of Health, announced in April 1991 plans for a women's health study. The study will examine the three major causes of death, disability, and frailty in women aged forty-five years and older: "cardiovascular diseases, cancers of the breast, lung, and colorectal tract, and osteoporosis" (Rosser and Woodson, 1992, p. 2).

Of these, cardiovascular diseases are the number one killer of older women of all racial/ethnic groups. Osteoporosis and the cancers are particularly problematic for older white women, although women from all racial/ethnic groups suffer from them to a certain extent. For example, while Black women experience a lower frequency of breast cancer, they also experience lower survival rates (64 percent) compared to white women (76 percent) (Avery, 1992).

It must be recognized as well that the diseases of major importance differ somewhat for women from various racial/ethnic groups. For Black, American Indian, and Hispanic women, diabetes and hypertension constitute major causes of death (Manley et al., 1985). For American Indian and Asian women, liver and stomach cancer, along with other cancers, are more prevalent than in other racial/ethnic groups. For Black and American Indian women, accidental deaths, including homicide, are significant (Manley et al., 1985). For example, in 1986 homicide was the leading cause of death for all Blacks age fifteen through thirty-five, including 19 of 1,000 African-American women (Avery, 1992). In addition, each racial/ethnic group may have particular health problems related to genetic disorders and syndromes such as sickle cell anemia and systemic lupus erythematosus in the Black population, and alpha- and beta-thalassemia, hemoglobin E disease, and hepatitis B in the Asian population, which need further funding and studying.

Since the mean and median ages of people of color, including women, are lower than those of the white population, the target age of forty-five for diseases causing death may be inappropriate for women of color. Ethnic minority women, with the possible exception of Asian women, experience relatively high rates of infant and maternal mortality. Alcoholism mortality in the American Indian female population is significantly higher than in the white population. American Indian women experience the highest proportion of alcohol deaths for men or women of any group (Finkelstein et al., 1990). The comparison of mortality rates from alcoholism of American Indian females in the age groups thirty-five to forty-four years, forty-five to fifty-four years, and fifty-five to sixty-four years from 1978 to 1980 were respectively 13.6, 8.5, and 7.3 times those of white females per 100,000 population. Using forty-five years as the cutoff eliminates significant numbers of women of color and their causes of death. AIDS also is increasing rapidly in young Black and Hispanic women. Now that women have begun to appear on the national health research agenda, care must be taken to ensure that white women and their concerns do not become the norm. Research on topics of importance for the health of women of color must also be included.

Women of color have become the target for particular aspects of women's health research. Often these areas represent issues of social concern or social problems. Using women of color as experimental subjects for such research identifies them with the social problem and suggests that its cause is linked to their inability to control their own bodies.

A current example of this type of research focuses on Black teenage pregnancy. Teenage pregnancy in the African-American population has recently received substantial funding and study (Dash, 1986; Avery, 1992). But as Patricia Hill Collins points out in her 1991 book *Black Feminist Thought*, the frequency of pregnancy among Black teenagers has actually declined. The rates that have increased are of pregnancy among white teenagers, and of births to both Black and white *unmarried* teenage women (Collins, 1991, p. 64). In 1993 the National Center for Health Statistics and the U.S. Census Bureau reported (Udansky, 1993) that 60 of every 1,000 teenage girls gave birth in 1990, up from 50 in 1986. Although overall birth rates remain highest among Black teens, rates rose fastest among Hispanics. "During the last half of the '80s, the rate went up 25 percent for Hispanics, 19 percent for whites and 12 percent for Blacks" (Udansky, 1993, 1A). In 1970, 31 percent of teen births were to unmarried mothers; in 1990 that figure was 68 percent. Identifying teen pregnancy with Black women and defining it as a medical problem that deserves research dollars and protocols helps educate the public about the very real medical issues (inadequate prenatal care, inappropriate nutrition, competition of growing mother and fetus for nutrients) that arise when children give birth to children. However, defining it as a medical problem may imply that social improvements such as more jobs, better education, and increased social services will do little to alleviate a problem with biological roots.

A second example which links women of color as research subjects with a social problem are the numerous current studies (Streissguth et al., 1991; Chasnoff, Landress, and Barrett, 1990; McCalla et al., 1991; Gillogley et al., 1990) to assess the prevalence of substance abuse during pregnancy. Several studies compared frequencies in clinic and private populations (Ney et al., 1990; Streissguth et al., 1991; Matera et al., 1990) or studied frequencies in inner-urban hospitals only (Gillogley et al., 1990). Clinics and inner-city hospitals, where the substance-abuse frequency was found to be higher, have higher proportions of patients who are women of color. This research helps to establish the baseline data which have led to laws such as that enacted by Florida mandating that physicians test and report women who they "suspect" may be using drugs or alcohol during pregnancy (Chasnoff, Landress, and Barrett, 1990).

Subsequent studies have revealed that Black women are almost ten times more likely to be tested and reported for drug use than white women (Chasnoff, Landress, and Barrett, 1990), and that 80 percent of cases brought against women for drug use during pregnancy have been against women of color (Pattrow, 1990). This research has redounded upon the overall health of pregnant women of color, who may avoid prenatal care if they use drugs or alcohol. The impact of adequate prenatal care on pregnancy outcome cannot be underestimated. Researchers agree that it is safer for a baby to be born to a drug-abusing, anemic, or diabetic mother who visits the doctor than to be born to a "normal" woman who does not (Pattrow, 1990; Johnson, 1987).

Definition of topics selected for research must be broadened to include problems which women of color experience as significant for their lives. While some topics such as teen pregnancy and substance abuse in pregnant women have been studied extensively, others continue to be under-studied and ignored. Domestic violence and violence in the communities in which they live and the rapid increase in AIDS have increased the death rate among Black and Hispanic women (Avery, 1992; Jenkins, 1992). Little research has examined the direct threat to women's health caused by these factors, or the toll that the stress from worrying about these issues, living in poverty, and enduring the sexism and racism of our society takes on women of color. Child abuse, sexual abuse, and incest, experienced by so many women in our society, must have priority on the research agenda for both women of color and white women.

APPROACHES AND METHODS

Choosing problems for research from the perspectives of women of color to include issues of importance as defined from their experience calls for rethinking approaches previously used for research on women's health.

Women of color should be included routinely in clinical trials for drug testing, and in all research protocols concerning any disease that occurs in women. In the past, women of color have typically been excluded because of their race or included without conscious consideration of their race in terms of its potential interaction with the disease under study.

Women of color have often been targeted for high-risk clinical trials, in which the drug under study was thought to have dangerous side effects. The initial testing of the birth control pill, which contained high doses of estrogen, carried out on 132 women in Puerto Rico before it was considered safe to market on the United States mainland (Zimmerman et al., 1980), is an example of such targeting.

As noted above, in some cases women of color have served as experimental subjects without their proper informed consent. Norma Jean Serena, an American Indian mother of three children, was the first individual to raise sterilization abuse as a civil rights issue. She charged that in 1970 health and welfare officials in Armstrong County, Pennsylvania, conspired to have her sterilized when her youngest child was delivered (Kelly, 1977). Ten Chicana women who spoke only Spanish sued the Los Angeles County Hospital for obtaining their consent in English for sterilization. Some were in labor at the time, others even under anesthesia. A few reported that they were told to sign the paper for relief of labor pains (Dreifus, 1975). More than one-third of women of childbearing age on the island of Puerto Rico were sterilized between 1940 and 1970 without their consent (Vasquez-Calzada, 1973). Goldzieher et al. (1971a, 1971b) gave placebos, without informing the recipients, to 76 poor, multiparous Chicana women at a San Antonio clinic who sought treatment to prevent further pregnancies, in experiments to investigate side effects such as nervousness and depression attributable to oral contraceptives. African-American women, American Indian women, and some lower-income white women have been forced to take birth control or be sterilized in order to receive government support for their children (Rodriguez-Trias, 1980).

Women of color have often been targeted for the receipt of dangerous drugs, uninformed participation in experiments, and coercion as victims of medical procedures they did not want (Rodriguez-Trias, 1980). Reversing that trend and convincing these women that the research they are now being asked to participate in is in their self-interest will be difficult.

Diversity within racial/ethnic groups as well as between groups can bias research results if it is not considered when selecting populations for health research. Recognition of ethnic/racial diversity among women of color and representation of that diversity in sample sizes proportionate to the racial/ethnic diversity in the United States population constitute the first steps toward studies more likely to yield accurate data. These steps may be insufficient without the recognition of other sources of diversity which significantly affect health.

Diversity within ethnic groups results from differences in economic class, sexual orientation, age, and other factors discussed elsewhere in this volume as common sources of diversity among women. Being a first-generation immigrant, having a language other than English as the primary language, or being unfamiliar with the health care system and accepted definitions of health and disease in the United States represent major sources of diversity within some ethnic/minority groups. These intragroup diversities, particularly those associated with first-generation immigrant status, often lead to significant, bipolar differences within racial/ethnic groups.

Asian-American women, for example, exhibit sharp discrepancies and bipolar patterns in their socioeconomic and health profiles (Manley et al., 1985). Certain subpopulations of Japanese-Americans, Chinese-Americans, and Korean-Americans immigrated to the United States during the nineteenth century. Most Asian-Americans from these groups tend to be well educated, speak English fluently, and enjoy relatively high socioeconomic status and good health. Some studies (Lin-Fu, 1983, 1984; Chinese Hospital Medical Staff and University of California School of Medicine, 1982) have examined the health and disease needs of these populations and provide limited baseline data for future studies.

In contrast, the majority of Asian/Pacific Americans are first-generation immigrants; many have arrived relatively recently as refugees from brutal political terror. This group of minorities (some of whom also come from China and Korea) encompass extreme diversity in language and cultures. In addition to socioeconomic deprivation and language and cultural barriers, many of these refugees and immigrants suffer from a high incidence of health problems (Manley et al., 1985). Reliance on folk remedies from their country of origin often complicates health by causing toxicity (Centers for Disease Control, 1983, 1984) and delaying the decision to seek Western medical care. No studies to date supply basic information or baseline data for this group.

Researchers who include Asian-American women in experimental protocols may obtain results about health and disease which are relatively useless if they fail to consider diversity with regard to immigrant status and socioeconomic, linguistic, and cultural factors within this racial/ethnic group. Because of the bipolar patterns in the socioeconomic and health status of first-generation immigrants compared to Asian-Americans born in this country, data such as means, medians, and modes based on such a combined sample of Asian-American women will not be representative of, or useful to, either group.

Similar difficulties arise when diversity within groups of American-Indian and Hispanic women is not considered in research design. For American Indian women, tribal differences, as well as differences based on living on reservations or in urban areas, have significant implications for their health. Socioeconomic differences, as well as immigration and political refugee patterns, among women from Central and Latin American countries complicate research on health in Hispanic women in ways similar to those among Asian-Americans. Failure to consider the full range of diversity—class, culture, immigrant status, language, education, age, sexual orientation—within each racial/ethnic group may compound bias in research methods.

Approaches that recognize diversity within racial/ethnic groups must be coupled with nontraditional methods to examine effectively health and disease in women of color. Cardiovascular disease, hypertension, diabetes, increasing rates of cancer, alcohol, and substance abuse, and infant and maternal mortality constitute the killers of all women; death rates are higher in women of color (Manley et al., 1985). In addition to the role of predisposing underlying genetic factors, their interaction with environmental and lifestyle factors determines the age of onset and severity of the disease.

None of these diseases can be adequately studied using the methods of any one traditional discipline (Hamilton, 1985). Interdisciplinary methods which combine approaches from the social and behavioral sciences with those of the biomedical and physical sciences are likely to reveal more complete information about these diseases for all people regardless of their race, gender, or class.

Poverty and stress have been linked to each of these killers. Poverty, with its accompanying inadequate access to health care and improper nutrition, and stress, also resulting from racism and sexism as experienced in our society, may partially explain the higher death rate among women of color from these killers. Studies designed to explore the causes and solutions for these diseases in women of color must consider the surrounding contexts of poverty and stress which initiate and enhance the progress of these diseases. Methods which fail to assess these factors will uncover only partial, biased information.

Data suggest that some of the causes for increased death rates among women of color have almost exclusively social origins. Four times as many Black women as white women die from homicide. Black maternal mortality rates are three times higher and the infant mortality rate is twice as high as that for white women (Manley et al., 1985). Homicide, domestic violence, and child abuse do not have biological causes. As the health care system redefines health and disease to include these aspects of physical violence, as well as sexual abuse and incest, research methods must also reflect this redefinition. Interdisciplinary methods, relying most heavily on qualitative approaches developed in some subareas of sociology, anthropology, and psychology, are likely to lead to more fruitful results for this research which is crucial to the lives of all women, particularly women of color.

THEORIES AND CONCLUSIONS DRAWN FROM THE DATA

Exclusion of women of color and their health care needs from clinical research has often resulted in inadequate or inappropriate theories and conclusions being drawn from the data. Clinicians and health care practitioners often translate this misinformation into practice when treating patients. In some cases, the lack of basic information leads to gross errors in diagnosing diseases, performing surgeries, and prescribing treatments. In other cases, stereotypes or inadequate information about sociocultural practices may result in less than optimal health care.

The absence of research and baseline data on some groups of women of color leaves practitioners without basic anatomical and genetic information necessary for diagnosis and treatment. For example, many health care providers are not aware that genetic disorders such as alpha- and beta-thalassemia, hemoglobin E disease, and glucose-6-phosphate dehydrogenase deficiency, as well as diseases such as hepatitis B and nasopharyngeal and stomach cancer, have a higher prevalence in certain subpopulations of Asian-Americans (Manley et al., 1985). The standard dosage of certain medications is often inappropriate for Asian/Pacific Americans, especially women, because of their smaller body size and weight, and certain surgical procedures may require modification for the same reason (Lin-Fu, 1984; Chinese Hospital Medical Staff, 1982).

The absence of basic information about the cultural definitions of health and disease and commonly used folk remedies may lead practitioners to misdiagnose and mistreat a disease. Recent immigrants, partially because of a lack of insurance and of familiarity with how to deal with the health care system, often rely on folk remedies. Some of those used by Asian immigrants have been reported as toxic. Specifically, traces of lead, arsenic, and mercury poisoning have been discovered and reported (Centers for Disease Control, 1983, 1984). Ignorance of cultural differences complicated by the use of folk remedies may delay diagnosis of the source of the illness by the practitioner.

Targeting women of color for certain types of research may cause clinicians to hold stereotypical views of women of color and particular diseases that limit accurate diagnosis. For example, numerous research studies have focused on sexually transmitted diseases in prostitutes in general (Centers for Disease Control, 1987; Cohen et al., 1988), and African-American women as prostitutes in particular (Centers for Disease Control, 1988). This may lead practitioners to hold a stereotyped view of African-American women. If an African-American woman goes to a health clinic, obstetrician-gynecologist, or emergency room complaining of stomach pain and/or flu-like symptoms, she is often assumed to have a sexually transmitted disease. Even if the woman swears that she is not sexually active, the practitioner may ignore symptoms suggestive of appendicitis or colitis to run more tests to find out which sexually transmitted disease she has. The opposite side of the stereotype is revealed when the practitioner fails to recognize a textbook case of secondary syphilis, including rash, because the woman presenting the symptoms is white, twenty-two years old, and a senior at a prestigious women's college (Gordon, 1977).

Several studies have also revealed that practitioners recognize and report at higher rates crack-cocaine abuse in African-American women and alcohol abuse in American Indian women compared to white women seeking prenatal care. In many cases these women lose their children after they are born or must serve jail time for detoxification. The American Civil Liberties Union reported that in forty-seven out of fifty-three cases brought against women for drug use during pregnancy in which the race of the woman was identifiable, 80 percent were brought against women of color (Pattrow, 1990, p. 2). Other studies have revealed that white middle-class women who use/abuse crack cocaine or alcohol during pregnancy are rarely reported and/or seldom risk losing their children. In March 1987, the state of Florida enacted legislation requiring that women known to have used drugs or alcohol during pregnancy be reported to health authorities. A study (Chasnoff, Landress, and Barrett, 1990) of the results of this mandated reporting revealed that although drug use by both private clients (13.1 percent) and public clients (16.3 percent) and white women (15.4 percent) and Black women (14.1 percent) was similar, Black women were almost ten times more likely to be tested and reported for drug use than white women; poor women using public health care facilities were more likely to be reported than affluent women able to afford private care. It is unclear whether the practitioner fails to recognize the abuse because the woman is white and middle-class or whether s/he simply fails to report it. In either case, the link between targeting African-American women for teen pregnancy and crack-cocaine research and American Indian women for fetal alcohol syndrome research and the reinforcement of stereotypical views held by practitioners seems likely.

Stereotyped views combined with research using methods that uncover only biological bases for health problems that in fact have both social and biological roots may lead practitioners to distance themselves from women of color and treat them inhumanely: sterilization of Puerto Rican women without informed consent (Vasquez-Calzada, 1973); forced sterilization of poor Hispanic or African-American women as a condition for receiving Medicaid (Rodriguez-Trias, 1980); giving Chicana women placebos without their knowledge when they sought contraception (Goldzieher et al., 1971a); coercion of HIV-positive African-American women to abort the fetuses they are carrying (Selwyn et al., 1989). Each of these practices represents inhumane treatment of patients by health care practitioners.

Undoubtedly these examples of inhumane treatment and countless other less overt coercions experienced by women of color every day at the hands of practitioners in our health care system have a variety of causes. The major causes in fact are probably not due to flaws in clinical research. However, some clinical research proposes only biological solutions for complex biological/social problems. For example, a biological solution such as Depo-Provera or Norplant implants (McLean, 1993) will be less effective in addressing teen pregnancy in Black females without accompanying strategies to raise self-esteem, increase education, and deal with underlying family dynamics. Stripped of the complex of social, economic, educational, and family dynamics issues that contribute to teen pregnancy, Norplant implants and Depo-Provera may prevent pregnancy in the short run and lead to the appearance of a solution for teen pregnancy. Without information about family planning, counseling to deal with dysfunctional families, and education and job skills, however, such approaches will not solve the basic problems causing teen pregnancy. These enforced biological solutions place control of the woman's body in the hands of the health care practitioner rather than the woman. This shift in control increases the power of the practitioner and decreases that of the woman. Some practitioners may forget the responsibility that such control entails and use that power for inhumane, coercive purposes. In this sense, flawed clinical research provides an atmosphere in which inhumane treatment seems less heinous.

The combination of racism and sexism has forced women of color to the periphery of the national health care agenda and the priorities for clinical research. Usually they and their health care needs have been ignored in traditional experimental studies. In a few cases, however, women of particular racial/ethnic groups have become the target for certain types of research. The focus of such research typically involves an aspect of reproduction in which a biological solution is sought for a complex medical/social problem. The bodies of women of color become the battleground over which control of this problem is fought.

The bipolarity surrounding health issues for women of color, in which they are either ignored or targeted, has biased research. The use of the white male as norm or his perspective concerning which health issues are important for women of color has determined the topics chosen for study, methods and approaches, and theories and conclusions drawn from the data.

The traditional research agenda must be changed to focus on the needs of women of color. Their own experiences should inform the determination of which issues are important and serve as the starting point for choosing topics for research. Using women of color and their needs as the central focus opens the door to different approaches to research, which may lead to the emergence of innovative practices to improve and sustain the health of women of color.

REFERENCES

Adisa, Opal Palmer. 1990. Rocking in the sun light: Stress and Black women. In Evelyn C. White (ed.), *The Black women's health book.* Seattle, Wash.: The Seal Press.

Alcena, Valiere. 1992. *The status of health of Blacks in the United States of America.* Dubuque, Iowa: Kendall/Hunt Publishing Co.

Avery, Byllye Y. 1992. The health status of Black women. In Ronald L. Braithwaite and Sandra E. Taylor (eds.), *Health issues in the Black community,* pp. 35–51. San Francisco: Jossey-Bass.

Boston Women's Health Book Collective. 1992. *The new our bodies, ourselves.* New York: Simon and Schuster.

Braithwaite, Ronald L., and Taylor, Sandra E. 1992. African-American health: An introduction. In Ronald L. Braithwaite and Sandra E. Taylor (eds.), *Health issues in the Black community,* pp. 3–5. San Francisco: Jossey-Bass.

Centers for Disease Control. 1983. Folk remedy associated lead poisoning in Hmong children. *Morbidity and Mortality Weekly Report* 32:505–506 (October 28).

———. 1984. Nonfatal arsenic poisoning in three Hmong patients. *Morbidity and Mortality Weekly Report* 33:347–349 (January 22).

———. 1987. Antibody to human immunodeficiency virus in female prostitutes. *Morbidity and Mortality Weekly Report* 36:157–161.

———. 1988. Distribution of AIDS cases by racial/ethnic group and exposure category, June 1, 1981–July 4, 1988. *Morbidity and Mortality Weekly Report* 37(SS-3):1–3.

Chase, Allan. 1977. *The legacy of Malthus: The social costs of the new scientific racism.* New York: Alfred Knopf.

Chasnoff, I. J.; Landress, H. J.; and Barrett, M. E. 1990. The prevalence of illicit drug or alcohol use during pregnancy and the discrepancies in mandatory reporting in Pinellas County. *New England Journal of Medicine* 322:1202–1206.

Chinese Hospital Medical Staff and University of California School of Medicine. 1982. Conference on health problems related to the Chinese in America. San Francisco, May 22–23.

Cohen, J., et al. 1988. Prostitutes and AIDS: Public policy issues. *AIDS and Public Policy Journal* 3:16–22.

Collins, Patricia Hill. 1991. *Black feminist thought.* New York: Routledge.

Dash, L. 1986. At risk: Chronicles of teenage pregnancy. *Washington Post,* January 26, pp. A1, A12, A13; January 27, pp. A1, A8, A9; January 28, pp. A1, A8, A9; January 29, pp. A1, A18; January 30, pp. A1, A14, A15; January 31, pp. A1, A16.

Dreifus, Claudia. 1975. Sterilizing the poor. *The Progressive* (December):13.

Finkelstein, Norma; Duncan, Sally Anne; Harman, Laura; and Smeltz, Janet. 1990. *Getting sober, getting well.* Cambridge, Mass.: Women's Alcoholism Program of CASPAR, Inc.

Gillogley, K. M.; Evans, A. T.; Hansen, R. L.; Samuels, S. J.; and Batra, K. K. 1990. The perinatal impact of cocaine, amphetamine, and opiate use detected by universal intrapartum screening. *American Journal of Obstetrics and Gynecology* 163:1535–1542.

Goldzieher, Joseph W.; Moses, Louis; Averkin, Eugene; Scheel, Cora; and Taber, Ben. 1971a. A placebo-controlled double-blind crossover investigation of the side effects attributed to oral contraceptives. *Fertility and Sterility* 22, no. 9:609–623.

———. 1971b. Nervousness and depression attributed to oral contraceptives: A double-blind, placebo-controlled study. *American Journal of Obstetrics and Gynecology* 22:1013–1020.

Gordon, Bonnie. 1977. Personal communication.

Gurwitz, Jerry H.; Nananda, F. Colonel; and Avorn, Jerry. 1992. The exclusion of the elderly and women from clinical trials in acute myocardial infarctions. *Journal of the American Medical Association* 11:1417.

Hamilton, Jean. 1985. Avoiding methodological biases in gender-related research. *Women's Health Report of the Public Health Service Task Force on Women's Health Issues.* Washington, D.C.: U.S. Department of Health and Human Services Public Health Service.

Jenkins, Bill. 1992. AIDS/HIV epidemics in the Black community. In Ronald L. Braithwaite and Sandra E. Taylor (eds.), *Health issues in the Black community*, pp. 55–63. San Francisco: Jossey-Bass.

Johnson, Elaine M. 1987. Women's health: Issues in mental health, alcoholism, and substance abuse. *Public Health Reports* (July/August):42–48.

Jones, Vida L. 1990. Lupus and Black women: Managing a complex chronic disability. In Evelyn C. White (ed.), *The Black women's health book.* Seattle, Wash.: The Seal Press.

Kelly, Joan. 1977. Sterilization and civil rights. *Rights* (publication of the National Emergency Civil Liberties Committee) (September/October).

Lin-Fu, J. S. 1983. Concerns and needs of Asian and Pacific American women (with focus on health). Address to the Montgomery County Commission for Women, Rockville, Md.

———. 1984. The need for sensitivity to Asian and Pacific Americans' health problems and concerns. Organization of Chinese American women speaks, July/August.

Manley, Audrey; Lin-Fu, Jane; Miranda, Magdalena; Noonan, Alan; and Parker, Tanya. 1985. Special health concerns of ethnic minority women in women's health. *Report of the Public Health Service Task Force on Women's Health Issues.* Washington, D.C.: U.S. Department of Health and Human Services.

Matera, C.; Warren, W. B.; Moomjy, M.; Fink, D. J.; and Fox, H. E. 1990. Prevalence of use of cocaine and other substances in an obstetric population. *American Journal of Obstetrics and Gynecology* 163:797–801.

McCalla, S., et al. 1991. The biologic and social consequences of perinatal cocaine use in an inner-city population: Results of an anonymous cross-sectional study. *American Journal of Obstetrics and Gynecology* 164:525–530.

McLean, Thomas. 1993. Requiring Norplant is coercive and bad idea. *The State* (April 1):12A.

Minkoff, Howard; Moreno, Jonathan; and Powderly, Kathleen. 1992. Fetal protection and women's access to clinical trials. *Journal of Women's Health* 1, no. 2:137–140.

Ney, J. A.; Dooley, S. L.; Keith, L. G.; Chasnoff, I. J.; and Sacol, M. L. 1990. The prevalence of substance abuse in patients with suspected preterm labor. *American Journal of Obstetrics and Gynecology* 162:1562–1567.

Pattrow, Lynn M. 1990. When becoming pregnant is a crime. *Criminal Justice Ethics* (Winter/Spring):41–47.

Pike, Marilyn. 1993. Systemic Lupus Erythematosus (SLE). Abstract published in *Journal of Women's Health* 2, no. 2:208.

Rodriguez-Trias, Helen. 1980. Sterilization abuse. In Rita Arditti, Pat Brennan, and Steve Cavrak (eds.), *Science and liberation*, pp. 113–127. Boston: South End Press.

Rosser, Sue V., and Woodson, Gayle. 1992. *The working group on research and research training needs of women and women's health issues at the National Institute on Deafness and Other Communication Disorders Report*. Bethesda, Md.: National Institutes of Health.

Selwyn, P. A., et al. 1989. Prospective study of human immunodeficiency virus infection and pregnancy outcomes in intravenous drug users. *Journal of the American Medical Association* 261:1289–1294.

Shulman, Lawrence E. 1985. Systemic lupus erythematosus. In *Women's Health Vol. II*, pp. 93–95. Public Health Service Task Force on Women's Health Issues. Washington, D.C.: U.S. Department of Health and Human Services.

Streissguth, A. P., et al. 1991. Cocaine and the use of alcohol and other drugs during pregnancy. *American Journal of Obstetrics and Gynecology* 164:1239–1243.

Udansky, Margaret L. 1993. Teen-age birth rates go back up. *USA Today*, May 14, pp. 1A, 7A.

Vasquez-Calzada, José. 1973. La Esterilizacion Femenina en Puerto Rico. *Revista de Ciencias Sociales* 17, no. 3 (San Juan):281–308.

White, Evelyn (ed.). 1990. *The Black women's health book*. Seattle, Wash.: The Seal Press.

Zimmerman, Bill, et al. 1980. People's science. In Rita Arditti, Pat Brennan, and Steve Cavrak (eds.), *Science and liberation*. Boston: South End Press.

CHAPTER SEVEN

Lesbians

Lesbian sexuality has been ignored in America. In both American history and the history of sexuality, the white, middle- to upper-class, heterosexual male has served as the norm against which the great men and great events which characterized most of history were measured. Political history and military history still employ this standard, and it continues to dominate historical research and teaching (Scott, 1988; Kelly-Gadol, 1975–76, 1979). Only relatively recently, led by the work of social historians such as Hareven (1974–75), Pleck (1978), Turbin (1979), Goldin (1977), and Fox-Genovese (1977), have women, working-class people, and people of color begun to be included in historical accounts.

Although considerable emphasis has been placed upon using the experience of these groups to recreate historical events from their perspective, the same norm is often used to situate or contrast with their perspective. Women's history or "herstory" (Scott, 1983) examines events from women's perspective to correct for the gender bias of the male perspective. Marxist, socialist, and other economic approaches correct for the class bias inherent in the "great men and great events" history told from the viewpoint of leaders representing the dominant class. African-American and other ethnic historians have been instrumental in including the stories of slaves and other racially oppressed groups in history. Even more recently (Katz, 1976), the field of gay history has emerged, as an attempt to correct for the heterosexual male perspective which has served as the mainline, traditional account of historical events.

As women and as nonheterosexuals, lesbians are doubly distanced from the heterosexual male norm. With some minor exceptions (Foster, 1956), lesbian history has been little studied until recently (Duggan, 1983; Sahli, 1979; Cruikshank, 1982; Faderman, 1977, 1979; Katz, 1976). Even the emergence of social history in contrast to white, male, heterosexual history overlooked lesbian history, which was lumped together with women's history or gay history.

HISTORY OF GROUPS OUTSIDE THE NORM

Early work in women's history tended toward what Gerda Lerner (1975) labeled compensatory history. Historians sought women who fit the great men (Scott, 1988), great events model. With the exception of gender, these women measured up to the usual white male norm. This compensatory approach corrected for the absence of women, while failing in most cases to consider diversity among women and continuing to repeat the errors of racial, class, and heterosexual bias. Compensatory history rarely challenged the conventional theories and approaches of history, as traditional research methods and paradigms were used to uncover these great women and their contributions to great events.

Even after scholars researching women's history discovered new methods that disclosed the lives of ordinary women and revealed racial and class diversity among women, lesbian history continued to be ignored. Just as compensatory history still used the male as norm as its guide for bringing great women to light, the models for research on diverse groups of women implicitly relied on a male as norm model. Marxist and economic approaches to history provided a satisfactory analysis of class for most men (Scott, 1987). Such analyses usually defined a woman's class by the class of her husband or father. Since the woman question in Marxism was never satisfactorily resolved (Goldman, 1931; Flax, 1981), many feminist critiques of Marxist approaches to history or Marxist critiques of women's history (Jaggar, 1983; I. Young, 1981) centered on the role of women in the family, on reproduction, and on possible discrepancies caused by interclass marriages. This focus did little to further issues of importance for lesbian history.

Similarly, African-American history and the histories of other racial groups defined themselves in contradiction to the white part of the white male, middle-class, heterosexual norm. African-American approaches often included Marxist analyses, since slavery and poverty meant that most African-Americans did not match the middle/upper-class aspect of the norm either. Scholars researching the history of Black women (Abrahams, 1975; Davis, 1971; Staples, 1973; Lerner, 1972) struggled to define this history not only in relationship to the white male norm but also in relationship to that of the Black male. The focus on the Black family and the friction between Black men and women (D. White, 1991) made it unlikely that scholars in African-American history would be leaders in lesbian history. The insistence in some Black history scholarship that homosexuality was a "white man's disease" never present in African cultures (Beam, 1986) steered many scholars of African-American culture away from examining the history of homosexuality in African-Americans. Since Black lesbians are triply distanced from the white, male, heterosexual norm, it is not surprising that very little research (Roberts, 1981; Hull et al., 1982; Hull, 1987; Smith, 1983; Shockley, 1983) has examined their lives.

Gay American history emerged in the 1970s (Katz, 1976) along with women's history, Black history, and the reemergence of socialist history. Recognizing another group whose voices and experiences were missing from the traditional accounts of history, scholars of gay history revealed the heterosexist bias and homophobia in such accounts. Since lesbians are often ignored by or are invisible to the rest of society, the volume of evidence documenting male homosexuality was substantially greater than that for lesbians. This dearth of evidence, combined with the fact that most of the first individuals undertaking the research were gay men, led the initial parameters for research and theories and conclusions drawn from the documents to be based on the gay male experience.

SEXUALITY IN HISTORY

Foucault (1980) brought the idea that sexuality is not repressed, but at the center of modern discourses, to the attention of historians. Sexuality has also traditionally been defined using a white, male, upper-middle-class, heterosexual norm. In contrast to the situation in some other cultures (Allen, 1986; Blackwood, 1984) and in previous historical periods (Bullough, 1976; Bullough and Voght, 1973; Crompton, 1980/81), women's sexuality in late nineteenth- and twentieth-century America was defined biologically. In addition to the central role given to procreation, Freud's "anatomy is destiny" (Freud, 1968, p. 18) characterized women's sexual development based upon what women lacked compared to the male norm.

Freud's use of the single concept of penis envy to explain the development of sexuality, normal gender development, and neurotic conflict in women (Person, 1990) was repudiated quickly by female psychoanalysts of the day. Horney (1924, 1926, 1932, 1933) challenged penis envy, ascribing femininity to female biology and awareness of the vagina, not disappointment over lacking a penis. Thompson (1950) suggested that the major sexual dilemma for women was not penis envy, but acknowledging their own sexuality in this culture. Other women (de Beauvoir, 1974) stated that what women envied was men's power, not their penis.

Freud did not ignore lesbian sexuality, but subsumed it under female heterosexuality as an immature state in which the woman failed to make the clitoral-to-vaginal transfer. Lesbian sexuality again was defined as doubly removed (first as female, then as failed heterosexual) from the male heterosexual norm.

Although male homosexuality has been accepted in some cultures (Blackwood, 1984; Duberman, Vicinius, and Chauncey, 1989; Bullough, 1976; Katz, 1976) or time periods as normal, as a higher form of sexual relationship than male heterosexuality, or as bisexuality, since the sixteenth century in America it has been defined in terms of deviation from the heterosexual male norm. In *Gay American History: Lesbians and Gay Men in the USA*, Katz delineates four periods in gay American history: homosexuality defined by theologians as a sin; by legislators as a legal problem or crime; by medical entrepreneurs as a biological anomaly; and finally by psychiatrists/psychologists as a psychic disturbance. Evidence of lesbianism can be found to correspond to each of these periods. Although not ignored, the history of lesbians is again defined against a male norm—that of the male homosexual. Lesbian history based on the experiences of lesbians, rather than as a subdiscipline within women's history or gay history, remains an understudied field which is only now beginning to emerge in its own right.

Application of these four temporal approaches to uncover lesbian sexual history leads to lesbian sexuality being either ignored or defined in terms of male homosexuality. For example, lesbian sexuality is never discussed in the Bible, although male homosexuality is discussed and the death penalty is prescribed for it in the Old Testament. Viewing homosexuality as a sin based on Biblical interpretations usually meant that lesbianism was ignored. However, some early evidence from Colonial records indicates that in 1636 the Reverend John Cotton of the Massachusetts Colonies recognized lesbian sexuality as sodomy and applied the same sanction of capital punishment to lesbian acts as to those of male homosexuals (Katz, 1976). In the later periods, legal and medical definitions and treatments for male homosexuality were frequently extended to lesbians, although sometimes in modified form. For example, in 1893 Dr. F. E. Daniel of Austin, Texas, proposed castration for male homosexuals and ovariectomy for lesbians to cure their sexual perversions (Katz, 1976). Lesbian sexuality is yet again doubly removed (first as homosexual, then as female) from the heterosexual male norm defining sexuality. Few studies have examined lesbian sexuality beginning from lesbian experience.

The history of lesbian sexuality serves as a paradigm for the approach to lesbians in other areas of their lives less directly related to their sexuality. Usually lesbianism is ignored, or overlooked, even when being a lesbian has implications for the issue under study. When lesbians are recognized, they are often subsumed as a subset of women or homosexuality where heterosexual females (Bernhard and Dan, 1986; Stevens and Hall, 1988) or homosexual males (Trippet and Bain, 1992) become the respective norms against which lesbians are measured. The implicit assumption underlying this failure to recognize health care issues for lesbians is either that lesbians do not exist, that they have precisely the same health care issues as heterosexual females, or in rare cases that they share the same health care issues as male homosexuals (Trippet and Bain, 1992). This ignoring or lumping together of lesbian health care issues becomes exacerbated by homophobia on the part of health care professionals. Not only does homophobia discourage lesbians from seeking necessary health care, but it also prevents health care workers from tying appropriate diagnoses and treatments to risk behaviors.

As discussed in the previous chapters, women's health in the United States has been defined against the white, middle-class, heterosexual male norm for research, diagnosis, and treatment of diseases. This definition is reflected in the exclusion of women from drug testing, the designation of some diseases which affect both sexes as male diseases, inadequate study of conditions specific to females, and disregard for women's experiences.

Given the lack of attention to women's health issues not directly related to procreation and sexual activity for heterosexual women, it is not surprising that virtually no research has explored lesbian health issues. Thought of as homosexuals and thus defined in opposition to their heterosexual counterparts, lesbians naturally become excluded from obstetrics/gynecology, the medical specialty devoted to women's health.

EFFECTS OF THE FAILURE TO STUDY LESBIAN HEALTH ISSUES

Very little research has included separate studies of health care issues for lesbians. The Santa Cruz Women's Health Collective (O'Donnell, 1977), the Radicalesbians Health Collective (1977), some women's health groups such as the National Women's Health Network, and some studies (Eliason, Donelan, and Randall, 1992; Robertson, 1992) have suggested differences in health and disease processes in lesbians and nonlesbians. For example, it is clear that lesbians have a much lower incidence of certain diseases such as cervical cancer. Heterosexual intercourse permits the transmission of the herpes, trichomoniasis, chlamydia, and human papilloma virus (HPV) thought to be major causes of cervical cancer. Beginning intercourse at an early age also increases the chances of cervical cancer (Boston Women's Health Book Collective, 1992). Cervical cancer is nonexistent in celibate women and rare in lesbians who have engaged in limited heterosexual intercourse or are not at risk from other factors such as DES exposure and smoking.

In contrast, lesbians may be at higher risk for certain other diseases such as breast and uterine cancer. Dr. Suzanne Haynes of the National Cancer Institutes estimates that one in three lesbians may develop breast cancer during her lifetime because lesbians are more likely than other women to fall into high-risk categories for the disease (Campbell, 1992). Women who have never had children are at an almost 80 percent greater risk for breast cancer than women who have had children; it may be inferred that lesbians are thus at increased risk because fewer lesbians have children than heterosexual women. Women with a higher body fat content have about a 55 percent greater risk of developing breast cancer; since overweight conditions are more acceptable in the lesbian community, this may present an additional risk factor for lesbians. Because of the need for Pap smears in order to receive birth control pills and a higher incidence of venereal diseases, heterosexually active women seek gynecological exams approximately every eight months. In contrast, lesbian women consult a gynecologist about every twenty-one months. Since gynecological exams include mammograms and breast examinations by physicians, lesbians are subject to these mechanisms for early detection of breast cancer at less frequent intervals than heterosexually active women (Campbell, 1992). These health factors, plus evidence that alcohol intake and smoking, factors which increase the risk of breast cancer, have been shown in some studies (Hall, 1992; Buenting, 1992) to be higher in lesbians than nonlesbians, led Haynes to theorize the one-in-three rate for breast cancer in lesbians (Campbell, 1992).

Despite these increased risks, no federal research dollars have targeted lesbian health issues as their focus of study. Even the newly initiated Office of Women's Health Research at the National Institutes of Health has not earmarked any of its $500 million Women's Health Initiative to undertake lesbian health research (Medical News and Perspectives, 1992).

Failure to identify and fund separate studies of lesbian health issues usually results in lesbians' being lumped together with heterosexual women in studies of women's health issues. Combining lesbians and heterosexual women may obscure not only the true incidence but also the cause of the disease. In addition to cervical cancer, the likelihood of most sexually transmitted diseases including gonorrhea, syphilis, herpes, and chlamydia being transmitted from males to females during hetero-sexual activity is dramatically greater than the likelihood of transmission from lesbian contact. Although transmission of such sexually transmitted diseases between lesbians does occur, the incidence is minuscule compared to transmission between male homosexuals, and to male-to-female and female-to-male transmission during heterosexual activities.

When lesbians are lumped together with heterosexual women in stud-ies of incidence and/or cause of sexually transmitted diseases or other gynecological problems from which they are exempt or for which they are at low risk because they do not engage in heterosexual intercourse, both lesbians and nonlesbians suffer. Defining such studies generally as research on "women's health issues" rather than on "health issues for women engaging in heterosexual sex" leads the general population and some health care workers to think that lesbians are at risk for diseases which they are unlikely to contract, while obscuring the true risk behavior for heterosexual women.

THE STATUS OF RESEARCH ON HOMOSEXUAL HEALTH

Even when lesbians are defined as homosexual, the norm for their health care issues continues to be the male. Lesbians are usually assumed to be a subset of or very similar to male homosexuals (Anderson, 1981; Corbett, Troiden, and Dodder, 1977; Hudson and Ricketts, 1980). Since male homosexuals are typically distinguished by their deviation from the male heterosexual norm, lesbians again find themselves at a double re-move. Lesbians are neither heterosexual nor male; thus their health issues continue to be overlooked or ignored. For example, most current funding for homosexual health care issues is directed toward the study of AIDS. Although lesbians tend politically to support the issue of funding AIDS for society in general, for male homosexuals, among whom the epidemic is rampant (Shilts, 1987), and heterosexual women, who represent the group in which AIDS is currently increasing most rapidly in the United States (Anastos and Marte, 1989), they receive few direct benefits of this research. Lesbians as a group engage in behaviors that put them at the lowest risk for contracting AIDS.

A related confusion arises when lesbians are not listed as a separate statistical category for frequency of diseases. The Centers for Disease Control does not include a separate category for lesbians in its groups for AIDS infection; homosexual men, bisexual men, and adult men are listed separately (Curran et al., 1988). Men not only are listed by sexual orientation but are further subdivided by intravenous drug use and race.

The statistics on all women collected by the CDC for HIV infection are not as complete as those collected for men. For example, no distinct category for women at double risk from infection as IV drug users and partners of infected men exists as it does for men. This may be responsible for the results suggesting that a significantly higher percentage of women (9 percent) than men do not understand the source of their AIDS infection (Anastos and Marte, 1989). This sloppy statistical reporting may lead to false complacency on the part of women who engage in heterosexual relations with men in which they may not be aware of their partner's risk-taking behavior.

The failure to separate out lesbians as a distinct group for statistics on AIDS leads the public to false understandings of the risk behaviors causing the disease. It may partially explain the common misunderstanding, even by 20 percent of nurse educators (Randall, 1989), that lesbians transmit AIDS. Lumping lesbians, celibate women, and heterosexually active women together obscures the increased risk of AIDS to women engaging in heterosexual activity, since lesbians and celibate women are at virtually no risk for AIDS from sexual activity. In a few cases female-to-female transmission has been suggested through an IV drug-using HIV-infected woman transmitting the virus through traumatic sex practices (Monzon and Capellan, 1987). Lesbians may also be vulnerable to HIV infection via artificial insemination from an infected donor as well as from blood transfusions.

This inappropriate lumping also reinforces the initial mistake made in research in this country when AIDS was designated by group rather than risk behaviors. The initial characterization of AIDS as a gay male disease, with the subsequent inclusion of IV drug users and Haitian immigrants, led to a plethora of problems resulting in lack of funding and study of AIDS and its transmission (Shilts, 1987) and diagnosis in many populations. This led the general public to believe that being a homosexual, rather than engaging in certain risk behaviors, causes AIDS.

Other health issues significant for the homosexual population may result in lesbians' receiving diagnosis and treatment that is less appropriate for them because the male has been chosen as the norm. Alcoholism, a problem for lesbians as well as male homosexuals, is thought to be underdiagnosed in the lesbian community. Some studies (Fifield, Latham, and Phillips, 1977; McKirnan and Peterson, 1989a, 1989b; Saghir and Robins, 1973) suggest that the drinking patterns of lesbians are more consistent with national norms for male drinkers than for female drinkers (Fifield, Latham, and Phillips, 1977; McKirnan and Peterson, 1989a, 1989b; McNally, 1989; Hall, 1992). Much of the study of alcoholism in homosexual populations has used the gay bar as a source for estimating and diagnosing the incidence of alcoholism (Hall, 1991). Limited research (Luly, 1991; Weathers, 1981) suggests that many lesbians, particularly in some geographic areas, such as the South, and from the upper and middle socioeconomic classes, may not frequent lesbian bars. This does not mean that they are not drinking elsewhere and may not be suffering from alcoholism. Similarly, the twelve-step treatment, the model considered to be most successful for treating alcoholics, was developed by two men using themselves (white, middle- to upper-class heterosexuals) as the norm. Feminists (Tallen, 1990; Muller, 1990; Hall, 1992) have critiqued the confrontational aspects of the model as less appropriate for many women who seek to avoid conflict. The self-revelation aspects of the model and involvement of the spouse in Al-Anon or co-dependents' groups are less appropriate for lesbians, who are likely neither to have a spouse nor to reveal much about their personal life in a lesbophobic society (Deevey and Wall, 1992). In some cases, AA is not sensitive to painful prior events such as rape, incest, battering, or other traumatic events for which alcohol or drug use becomes a symptom (Hall, 1992).

The use of the white heterosexual male as the norm for health care issues has resulted in a lack of information about the health and disease processes of lesbians. The information available often comes from inappropriate extrapolation from the female heterosexual or male homosexual population to the lesbian. The main people damaged by this lack of information are lesbians. Being ignored has led them in turn to ignore themselves with regard to some crucial health care issues. Ironically, lesbians' being ignored or subsumed under "women's" or "homosexuals'" health issues also hurts nonlesbians, especially heterosexual women, who then fail to understand the significance of risk behaviors or lifestyle choices for health and disease processes.

HEALTH CARE ISSUES DEFINED BY LESBIANS

Inappropriate inclusion of lesbians in studies of and statistics on women's health problems, such as cervical cancer, and homosexual health problems, such as AIDS, has consequences beyond obscuring the true risk behavior causing these diseases. It also means that health issues as defined from lesbian experience have not been explored. The absence of this focus implies that research on health issues important to lesbian women, and which may be increasingly important for elderly, widowed, or celibate heterosexual women, whose health can no longer appropriately be defined around procreation and heterosexual activity, has not been undertaken. For example, studies of ways to diagnose endometriosis in women not engaging in heterosexual intercourse or trying to become pregnant may reveal new information about the symptoms of endometriosis. An examination of the effects of bodybuilding, karate, and self-defense in helping women to ward off attacks and battering may be as important for women's health as contraception. As more funds are allocated to the formerly neglected aspects of menopause, attention to the models of communities of women living together as they age may be more important than studies of the empty nest syndrome in a society where many women have few children and the aging population is primarily female.

LESBIANS AS A MODEL

Overlooking lesbians in research design ignores the possibility that the lesbian may be the best model for exploring some aspects of women's health. In their attempts to find self-definition and to reject many of the definitions and needs projected onto them by the surrounding culture, lesbians have become aware that most institutions use the white, middle-class, heterosexual male as the norm. They have struggled to define themselves in a patriarchal culture by asking what their own experience has been and what their needs are. This struggle provides them with a beginning for a female-centered model of health care. Lesbians and the lesbian community seek alternatives to male-focused systems. Health care research in which the health and disease processes of women's bodies are examined without a focus on contraception, sexually transmitted diseases, pregnancy, childbirth, and accommodation of sexual functions to fit men's needs would open the door to a model for women's health and disease free from the gynecological complications normally imposed by heterosexual activity. This model would provide baseline data for normal health events such as menarche, menopause, and aging, as well as disease processes, in the absence of reproductive complications. Applicable particularly to lesbians, it would also apply well to the large numbers of celibate and heterosexual women without children.

Ignoring lesbians in general in research designs and discussions of health issues overlooks and obscures particular diversities among lesbians. With the exception of their sexual orientation, lesbians demonstrate as much variety with regard to race, class, occupation, and age as their heterosexual sisters. Indeed, many lesbians also share a history of heterosexual experiences. Many married, either before they recognized their sexual orientation or as an attempt to conform to the pressures for compulsory heterosexuality in this society. Many lesbians are biological parents, their children having been conceived during a heterosexual relationship or through artificial insemination. Studies using lesbians must pay attention to these diverse factors and their implications for health in order to avoid the similar confounding among variables which occurs when lesbians are lumped together with heterosexual women or male homosexuals.

DIVERSITY AMONG LESBIANS

Attention to lesbians as a group and the diversity among them (West, 1987; Gomez and Smith, 1990) should lead to cleaner research designs with less conflation of variables. For example, a study of lesbians who have never had heterosexual sex compared with those who have for varying lengths of time might definitively establish the duration of heterosexual activity correlated with cervical cancer.

Rethinking the differences among lesbians also reveals situations when sexual orientation should not be used to distinguish among women. For example, to study the role of childbearing in preventing breast cancer, childless lesbians should be grouped with childless heterosexual, bisexual, or celibate women for comparison with women from those groups who have borne children. Similarly, studies of cervical cancer should combine heterosexual and lesbian women who have never had intercourse for comparison with women who have had intercourse regardless of their present sexual orientation. This attention to diversity shifts the focus from inappropriate groups to risk behaviors.

Some lesbians may have more difficulty than others in dealing with their sexual orientation in this homophobic society. This may have direct effects on health care research, particularly research based in clinical or case data (Swanson et al., 1972). Extant literature on lesbian health, particularly mental health, is likely to include an overrepresentation of lesbians who have problems (Morin, 1977; Stevens, 1992). Their representation in the literature as lesbians in many cases reflects some disclosure (through self or referral) that lesbianism is perceived as part of or related to their health problem.

Overexamination of and research centered on the lesbian population seeking or referred for counseling and therapy has possibly led to misperceptions about the prevalence and severity of problems that sexual orientation causes for lesbians (Freedman, 1975; Smith, Johnson, and Guenther, 1985; Stevens and Hall, 1988). Since lesbians having fewer problems tend not to seek help, they are underrepresented in the literature or unknowingly lumped together with heterosexual women. Presumably this pattern of overrepresentation of lesbians with problems and underrepresentation of those without holds for other aspects of health as well. Thus health care practitioners and the general population are provided with a false picture of the prevalence of diseases and difficulties in the lesbian population.

STRESS IN LESBIANS

The overrepresentation/underrepresentation dilemma may also obscure the contributions of social and psychological factors to physical disease processes. The role that stress plays in cardiovascular disease, ulcers, skin allergies, lupus, and even cancer, for example, has been well documented (Selye, 1956; Haynes and Feinleib, 1980). Although most lesbians view their sexual orientation as a positive force in their lives, many would admit that being a lesbian in a homophobic society is quite stressful (Underhill and Ostermann, 1991), particularly for lesbians of color who fight racism and sexism (Lorde, 1984; Smith, 1983). The role that this stressor, in comparison to others, plays in diseases more prevalent in the lesbian population needs to be studied. In order to evaluate this role, a lesbian population needs to be clearly identified, and interdisciplinary methods from the social sciences and natural sciences need to be utilized to elucidate the relationship between stress and disease in lesbian lives.

Jean Hamilton has called for interactive models that draw on both the social and natural sciences to explain complex problems:

> Particularly for understanding human, gender-related health, we need more interactive and contextual models that address the actual complexity of the phenomenon that is the subject of explanation. One example is the need for more phenomenological definitions of symptoms, along with increased recognition that psychology, behavioral studies, and sociology are among the "basic sciences" for health research. Research on heart disease is one example of a field where it is recognized that both psychological stress and behaviors such as eating and cigarette smoking influence the onset and natural course of a disease process. (1985, IV-62)

Such interdisciplinary methods might be useful for studying the role of stress in various diseases in the lesbian population.

INTERACTIONS BETWEEN LESBIANS AND HEALTH CARE PROFESSIONALS

Ignoring lesbian health issues in research has led to inappropriate diagnoses and treatments for lesbians. For many health care practitioners, the absence of lesbians as a group from studies and discussions has been translated into the assumption that no lesbians seek health care services or that heterosexual activity should be assumed for all patients. In fact, a significant issue hindering many lesbians from seeking health care is homophobia or insensitivity on the part of health care practitioners.

HOMOPHOBIA AND HEALTH CARE PROFESSIONALS

Historically within this century, lesbians have been characterized by the medical profession as sick, dangerous, aggressive, tragically unhappy, deceitful, contagious, and self-destructive (Bergler, 1957; Caprio, 1954; Romm, 1965; Socarides, 1968; Wilbur, 1965; Wolff, 1971). Defined as a disease at the turn of the century, lesbianism was characterized by health care professionals until the early 1980s through an emphasis upon etiology, diagnosis, and cure (Morin, 1977; Schwanberg, 1985, 1990; Watters, 1986).

Not surprisingly, many health care professionals hold extremely homophobic attitudes, which are reflected in their interactions with and diagnoses and treatments of lesbian patients. In a recent review of research related to lesbians' experiences with health care during the past twenty years, Stevens (1992) discovered nine studies about health care providers' attitudes toward lesbian clients. All nine studies (Levy, 1978; Liljestrand, Gerling, and Saliba, 1978; Garfinkle and Morin, 1978; T. A. White, 1979; Douglas, Kalman, and Kalman, 1985; Mathews et al., 1986; E. W. Young, 1988; Randall, 1989; and Eliason and Randall, 1991) uncovered significant homophobic attitudes among health care professionals. Particularly revealing are relatively recent studies. A 1986 (Mathews et al.) convenience sample of 1,000 M.D.'s in San Diego found that 23 percent were severely homophobic; surgeons, gynecologists, and family practice M.D.'s were most homophobic. This same study demonstrates the direct effects of these attitudes on their treatment of gay and lesbian clients: 40 percent were uncomfortable with treating gays and lesbians; 30 percent opposed admitting gays and lesbians to medical schools; 40 percent would not refer clients to gay or lesbian colleagues (Mathews et al., 1986). A 1988 study (Young) of nurses uncovered the fact that 64 percent of RNs hold negative attitudes such as pity, disgust, unease, embarrassment, fear, and sorrow toward gays and lesbians; 50 percent of RNs with these feelings stated that they had no desire to change (Young, 1988). Studies of nursing educators (Randall, 1989) and nursing students (Eliason and Randall, 1991) reveal similar homophobic attitudes which are correlated with medical misinformation, such as the belief of 20 percent of nursing educators (Randall, 1989) and 28 percent of students (Eliason and Randall, 1991) that lesbians transmit AIDS.

Lesbians directly experience the homophobic attitudes of health care professionals. These experiences range from an assumption of heterosexuality on the part of the health care provider (Dardick and Grady, 1980; Johnson and Palermo, 1984; Reagan, 1981; Stevens and Hall, 1988) through a negative reaction (72 percent of respondents) when patients disclosed their sexual preference (Stevens and Hall, 1988) to attempts to cure their lesbianism (Glascock, 1981, 1983).

Most lesbians believe their health care would be of higher quality if they could safely disclose their sexual identity (Hume, 1983; Smith, Johnson, and Guenther, 1985; Cochran and Mays, 1988; Stevens and Hall, 1988, 1990). However, the majority (Hume, 1983; Olesker and Walsh, 1984; Glascock, 1981, 1983; Cochran and Mays, 1988) do not disclose because of fears and experiences of mistreatment, intimidation, humiliation, and lack of safety in health care interactions (Stevens, 1992).

Inability to disclose their sexual orientation, coupled with the negative reactions they are confronted with when they do, leads many lesbians to delay seeking health care (Bradford and Ryan, 1988; Deevey, 1990; Stevens and Hall, 1988; Zeidenstein, 1990). Distrusting mainstream health care (Deevey, 1990), many lesbians are more likely to seek help for a health problem from lesbian friends than from the health care system (Saunders, Tupac, and MacCulloch, 1988), or to seek referral from a friend to a supportive health care professional. In addition to the fact that their needs are not being met, a 1992 study revealed other reasons lesbians do not seek health care from traditional sources: "(a) low-cost, natural, or alternative care is not provided; (b) holistic care is not provided; (c) little preventive care and education are provided; (d) communication and respect are lacking; and (e) few women-managed clinics are available" (Trippet and Bain, 1992, p. 148).

Assuming a heterosexual orientation (Glascock, 1981, 1983; Stevens and Hall, 1988), many obstetricians/gynecologists routinely begin examinations of women aged sixteen to fifty-five by asking questions about the kind of contraception used and whether it is working successfully. They require all of their patients to have yearly Pap smears, without first ascertaining whether or not the woman is at risk for cervical cancer. A yearly Pap smear may be a waste of time and money for a woman who has never engaged in heterosexual intercourse or other behaviors that put her at risk for cervical cancer.

Because of the assumption by most health care practitioners of the heterosexual norm, many lesbians and celibate women refuse routine examinations or delay seeking treatment for serious symptoms (Bradford and Ryan, 1988; Deevey, 1990; Stevens and Hall, 1988; Zeidenstein, 1990) because they find the questions about contraception and heterosexual activity to be distasteful. Diseases such as endometriosis are unlikely to be diagnosed in lesbians if the practitioner uses pain during intercourse as the major criterion. Some lesbians fear that revealing their sexual orientation to a health care practitioner may lead to loss of jobs or children if this information is recorded in medical records which may become available to employers or social service workers (Glascock, 1981, 1983; Hume, 1983; Stevens and Hall, 1988, 1990).

LESS HOMOPHOBIC APPROACHES FOR PRACTITIONERS

Health care practitioners may avoid some of this discomfort and fear (as well as educating all of their patients to varieties of sexual orientation) by presenting different health risks for different groups. A practitioner might begin an initial, general examination by indicating that depending upon the patient's sexual activities, she may be at risk for different health problems. For example, if she is currently engaging in heterosexual intercourse and does not wish to become pregnant, she should use some contraceptive device. Prevention of sexually transmitted diseases, including AIDS, is likely to be an issue for her, depending upon the nature of her relationship with her partner(s). She should definitely have a yearly

Pap smear. If she has never engaged in heterosexual intercourse and is not planning to do so in the near future, contraception and yearly Pap smears are not necessary for her unless she has other risk factors such as being a DES daughter. It is also less likely that she will need protection against sexually transmitted diseases (STDs). If she did engage in heterosexual intercourse in the past, but is not doing so now and does not plan to in the near future, then contraception and STD prevention may not be an issue for her, but she should have a Pap smear now and at three-year intervals.

Similar approaches might be taken for discovering whether or not the woman has had children and the risks this poses for breast cancer, uterine cancer, and endometriosis. This approach does not assume a heterosexual or a lesbian norm. It educates the patient about risk behaviors that may lead to increased incidence of certain diseases, thus providing her with more accurate information. It also educates the public about diversity with regard to sexual orientation in the population. In order for a practitioner to use this approach, s/he must be educated to recognize that lesbians do exist and to be knowledgeable about their health issues.

Public health campaigns to educate women about health promotion and disease prevention need to be oriented toward risk behaviors with the recognition that women have diverse sexual orientations. Public service announcements which encourage every woman to have an annual Pap smear do not focus on risk behaviors. They assume that all women engage in heterosexual activity and inadequately convey to the public the risk behavior responsible for cervical cancer. These announcements repeat for public information the initial mistakes in research design which define women in relationship to sexual activity with men.

Even when health care practitioners are aware that lesbians exist, they may not recognize the diversity among them. Assumptions of stereotypes, partially derived from medical literature (Morin, 1977), that lesbians dress in more masculine clothing, hold certain occupations, or exhibit "butch" mannerisms, may lead health care practitioners to think that they can spot a lesbian and modify their questions and examination for the health care issues for which she is at risk. Since lesbians exhibit considerable variation with regard to race, occupation, mode of dress, appearance, history of previous sexual activity, and pregnancy, ignoring their diversity may also lead to inappropriate treatment and diagnosis. Asking questions to reveal risk factors rather than assuming a norm for heterosexuality or lesbianism is the only way to ensure accurate diagnosis and appropriate treatment.

When a woman does reveal her sexual orientation to the health care practitioner, s/he must be cautious not to assume that this automatically means that the woman engages in a particular risk behavior. Risk behaviors such as anal intercourse, not homosexuality itself, put male homosexuals at risk for HIV. Similarly, not engaging in heterosexual or anal intercourse, not simply current sexual orientation, puts lesbians at less risk for cervical cancer or AIDS than women who engage in those activities.

A major reason that AIDS has reached epidemic proportions in the United States was the initial mistake made in identifying groups rather than specific risk behaviors not tied to sexual orientation. The campaign against AIDS has been relatively less successful in the Hispanic community. Although multiple reasons exist for the failure, a substantial factor is that the prevention campaign described as risky sexual practices often used by male homosexuals or bisexuals. Many Hispanic men who engage in anal sex with other men do not identify that behavior as a "sexual practice used by male homosexuals or bisexuals." Since these men also engage in heterosexual intercourse with their wives and/or girlfriends, they do not consider themselves to be homosexual or bisexual. As health care practitioners recognize lesbianism and help to define and educate themselves and the public about lesbian health care issues, they must take care to avoid similar problems of labeling by group rather than describing behaviors.

Describing specific risk behaviors rather than ascribing them to lesbians because of their sexual orientation will open the way to a better understanding of lesbian health care issues without reinforcing the status quo of ignorance and oppression from homophobia. The current condition of ignoring lesbians and their health care needs must not continue. It is tragic for lesbians who remain ignorant about their own health care issues; health care practitioners and the nonlesbian population also suffer. When lesbians are ignored in research design, it may lead to their inappropriate inclusion or exclusion from studies of health issues; this obscures the true incidence and cause of some diseases for both lesbian and nonlesbian women. Inappropriate inclusion or exclusion from populations sampled may be translated into inaccurate diagnosis and treatment. Precious resources may be unnecessarily wasted in overprescribing tests such as Pap smears and tests for STDs.

As women's health initiatives are being brought to the fore and as more money is targeted for study of women's health issues, lesbians must be recognized as a group with significant and understudied health needs. Lesbians have fought for funding and study of women's health in general. Homosexuals have demonstrated limited success in obtaining funding for study of diseases such as AIDS that have a significant impact on the health of male homosexuals. Many lesbians have joined their homosexual brothers in fighting homophobia about AIDS, caring for AIDS patients, and bringing political pressure for AIDS research dollars. Male homosexuals must also join lesbians in recognizing that health issues for lesbians represent another facet of homosexual health that deserves attention.

Previously defined by the male, heterosexual norm, both women in general and male homosexuals have struggled for their own health agendas and should be understanding of the need for lesbians to define their own health needs. Lesbian health needs cannot be defined exclusively by either women's health needs or homosexual health needs. Overlapping both groups in many respects, but separate from each in some respects, lesbians are women with a homosexual orientation. Lesbian health issues deserve study and definition based on lesbian experience.

REFERENCES

Abrahams, R. D. 1975. Negotiating respect: Patterns of presentation among black women. *Journal of American Folklore* 88:58–80.

Allen, Paula G. 1986. Lesbians in American Indian cultures. In *The Sacred Hoop*, pp. 106–117. Boston: Beacon Press.

Anastos, K., and Marte, C. 1989. Women—the missing persons in the AIDS epidemic. *Health PAC Bulletin* 19, no. 4:6–13.

Anderson, C. L. 1981. The effect of a workshop on attitudes of female nursing students toward male homosexuality. *Journal of Homosexuality* 7:57–69.

Arditti, Rita; Duelli Klein, Renate; and Minden, Shelley. 1984. *Test-tube women: What future for motherhood?* London: Pandora Press.

Beam, J. (ed.). 1986. *In the life: A Black gay anthology*. Boston: Alyson.

Bergler, E. 1957. *Homosexuality: Disease or a way of life?* New York: Hill and Wang.

Bernhard, Linda, and Dan, Alice. 1986. Redefining sexuality from women's own experiences. *Nursing Clinics of North America* 21:123–136.

Blackwood, E. 1984. Sexuality and gender in certain native American tribes: The case of the cross-gender female. *Signs* 10:27–42.

Boston Women's Health Book Collective. 1992. *The new our bodies, ourselves: Updated and expanded for the 90's*. New York: Simon and Schuster.

Bradford, J., and Ryan, C. 1988. *The national lesbian health care survey*. Washington, D.C.: National Lesbian and Gay Health Foundation.

Buenting, Julie A. 1992. Health life-styles of lesbian and heterosexual women. *Health Care for Women International* 13, no. 2:165–173.

Bullough, V. 1976. *Sexual variance in society and history*. New York: John Wiley.

Bullough, Vern, and Voght, M. 1973. Homosexuality and its confusion with the "Secret Sin" in pre-Freudian America. *Journal of the History of Medicine* 28, no. 2:143–154.

Campbell, Kristina. 1992. 1 in 3 lesbians may get breast cancer, expert theorizes. *The Washington Blade*, October 2, pp. 1, 23.

Caprio, F. S. 1954. *Female homosexuality: A psychodynamic study of lesbians*. New York: Citadel.

Cochran, S. D., and Mays, V. M. 1988. Disclosure of sexual preference to physicians by Black lesbian and bisexual women. *Western Journal of Medicine* 149:616–619.

Corbett, S. L.; Troiden, R. R.; and Dodder, R. A. 1977. Tolerance as a correlate of experience with stigma: The case of the homosexual. *Journal of Homosexuality* 3:3–13.

Corea, G., et. al. (eds.). 1987. *Man-made women: How new reproductive technologies affect women*. Bloomington: Indiana University Press.

Corea, G., and Ince, S. 1987. Report of a survey of IVF clinics in the USA. In Patricia Spallone and Deborah L. Steinberg (eds.), *Made to order: The myth of reproductive and genetic progress*. Oxford: Pergamon Press.

Cowan, Belinda. 1980. Ethical problems in government-funded contraceptive research. In Helen Holmes, Betty Hoskins, and Michael Gross (eds.), *Birth control and controlling birth: Women-centered perspectives*, pp. 37–46. Clifton, N.J.: Humana Press.

Crompton, L. 1980/81. The myth of lesbian impunity: Capital laws from 1270 to 1791. *Journal of Homosexuality* 6, nos. 1/2:11–25.

Cruikshank, Margaret (ed.). 1982. *Lesbian studies: Present and future*. New York: Feminist Press.

Curran, J. W., et al. 1988. Epidemiology of HIV infection and AIDS in the United States. *Science* 239:610–616.

Dardick, L., and Grady, K. E. 1980. Openness between gay persons and health professionals. *Annals of Internal Medicine* 93:115–119.

Davis, A. 1971. Reflections on the Black woman's role in the community of slaves. *Black Scholar* 3:7.

de Beauvoir, Simone. 1974. *The second sex*. Trans and ed. H. M. Parshley. New York: Vintage Books.

Deevey, S. 1990. Older lesbian women: An invisible minority. *Journal of Gerontological Nursing* 16, no. 5:35–39.

Deevey, Sharon, and Wall, Lana. 1992. How do lesbian women develop serenity? *Health Care for Women International* 13, no. 2:199–208.

Douglas, C. J.; Kalman, C. M.; and Kalman, T. P. 1985. Homophobia among physicians and nurses: An empirical study. *Hospital and Community Psychiatry* 36:1309–1311.

Dreifus, Claudia. 1978. *Seizing our bodies*. New York: Vintage Books.

Duberman, M.; Vicinius, M.; and Chauncey, G. Jr. 1989. *Hidden from history: Reclaiming the gay and lesbian past*. New York: NAL Books.

Duggan, L. 1983. The social enforcement of heterosexuality and lesbian resistance on the 1920's. In A. Swedlow and A. Lessinger (eds.), *Class, race, and sex: The dynamics of control*, pp. 75–92. Boston: G. K. Hall.

Ehrenreich, Barbara, and English, Deirdre. 1978. *For her own good*. New York: Anchor Press.

Eliason, M. J., and Randall, C. E. 1991. Lesbian phobia in nursing students. *Western Journal of Nursing Research* 13:363–374.

Eliason, Michele; Donelan, Carol; and Randall, Carla. 1992. Lesbian stereotypes. *Health Care for Women International* 13, no. 2:131–144.

Faderman, Lillian. 1977. Emily Dickinson's letters to Sue Gilbert. *Massachusetts Review* 18, no. 2:197–225.

———. 1979. Who hid lesbian history? *Frontiers* 4, no. 3:74–75.

Fifield, L. H.; Latham, D. J.; and Phillips, C. 1977. *Alcoholism in the gay community: The price of alienation, isolation and oppression*. Los Angeles: Gay Community Services Center.

Flax, J. 1981. Do feminists need Marxism? In *Building feminist theory: Essays from "Quest," A feminist Quarterly*, pp. 174–185. New York: Longman.

Foster, Jane. 1956. *Sex variant women in literature*. New York: Vantage.

Foucault, Michel. 1980. *The history of sexuality*. Vol. I: *An Introduction*. New York: Vintage.

Fox-Genovese, Elizabeth. 1977. Property and patriarchy in classical bourgeois political theory. *Radical History Review* 4:36–59.

Freedman, M. 1975. Homosexuals may be healthier than straights. *Psychology Today* (March).

Freud, Sigmund. 1968. The passing of the Oedipus complex. In Sigmund Freud, *Sexuality and the psychology of love*. New York: Collier Books.

Garfinkle, E. M., and Morin, S. F. 1978. Psychologists' attitudes toward homosexual psychotherapy clients. *Journal of Social Issues* 34, no. 3:101–112.

Glascock, Eleanor L. 1981. *Access to the traditional health care system by nontraditional women: Perceptions of a cultural interaction*. Paper presented at the annual meeting of the American Public Health Association, Los Angeles, November.

———. 1983. *Lesbians growing older: Self-identification, coming out, and health concerns.* Paper presented at the annual meeting of the American Public Health Association, Dallas, November.

Goldin, C. 1977. Female labor force participation: The origin of black and white differences, 1870 and 1880. *Journal of Economic History* 37:87–108.

Goldman, Emma. 1931. *Living my life.* Vol. 2. New York: Alfred A. Knopf. Reprint. New York: Dover Publications, 1970.

Gomez, J., and Smith, B. 1990. Taking the home out of homophobia: Black lesbian health. In Evelyn C. Hite (ed.), *The Black women's health book: Speaking for ourselves,* pp. 198–213. Seattle, Wash.: Seal Press.

Grobbee, D. E., et al. 1990. Coffee, caffeine, and cardiovascular disease in men. *New England Journal of Medicine* 321:1026–1032.

Hall, Joanne M. 1991. *Lesbians and alcohol: Patterns and paradoxes in medical notions and lesbian beliefs.* Manuscript submitted for publication.

———. 1992. An exploration of lesbians' images of recovery from alcohol problems. *Health Care for Women International* 13, no. 2:181–198.

Hamilton, Jean. 1985. Avoiding methodological biases in gender-related research. In *Women's health report of the Public Health Service Task Force on Women's Health Issues.* Washington, D.C.: U.S. Department of Health and Human Services Public Service.

Hareven, T. 1974–75. Family time and industrial time: Family and work in a planned corporation town, 1900–1924. *Journal of Urban History* 1:365–389.

Haynes, S. G., and Feinleib, M. 1980. Women, work and coronary heart disease: Prospective findings from the Framingham heart study. *American Journal of Public Health* 70, no. 2:133–141.

Holmes, Helen B., et al. (eds.). 1980. *Birth control and controlling birth: Women centered perspectives.* Clifton, N.J.: The Humana Press.

Horney, Karen. 1924. On the genesis of the castration complex in women. *International Journal Psychoanalysis* 5:50–65.

———. 1926. The flight from womanhood: The masculinity-complex in women, as viewed by men and by women. *International Journal Psychoanalysis* 7:324–339.

———. 1932. The dread of women: Observations on a specific difference in the dread felt by men and by women respectively for the opposite sex. *International Journal Psychoanalysis* 13:348–360.

———. 1933. The denial of the vagina: A contribution to the problem of the genital anxieties specific to women. *International Journal Psychoanalysis* 14:57–70.

Hubbard, Ruth. 1990. *Politics of women's biology.* New Brunswick, N.J.: Rutgers University Press.

Hudson, W. W., and Ricketts, W. A. 1980. A strategy for the measurement of homophobia. *Journal of Homosexuality* 5:357–372.

Hull, Gloria T. 1987. Alice Dunbar Nelson and Angela Wild Grimke. In *Color, sex, and poetry: Three women writers of the Harlem Renaissance,* pp. 33–104. Bloomington: Indiana University Press.

Hull, Gloria T.; Scott, Patricia B.; and Smith, Barbara (eds.). 1982. *All the women are white, all the Blacks are men, but some of us are brave: Black women's studies.* New York: Feminist Press.

Hume, B. J. 1983. Perspectives on women's health: Disclosure decisions, needs, and experiences of lesbians. Unpublished master's thesis, Yale University.

Jaggar, Alison M. 1983. *Feminist politics and human nature.* Totowa, N.J.: Rowman and Allanheld.

Johnson, S., and Palermo, J. 1984. Gynecological care for the lesbian. *Clinical Obstetrics and Gynecology* 27:724–730.

Katz, Jay N. 1976. *Gay American history: Lesbians and gay men in the USA.* New York: Meridien. Revised ed. 1992.

Kelly-Gadol, J. 1975–76. The social relations of the sexes: Methodological implications of women's history. *Signs* 1:816.

Kelly-Gadol, Joan. 1979. The doubled vision of feminist history: A postscript to the "Woman and Power" Conference. *Feminist Studies* 5:216–227.

Kirschstein, Ruth L. 1985. *Women's health: Report of the Public Health Service Task Force on Women's Health Issues.* Vol. 2. Washington, D.C.: U.S. Department of Health and Human Services Public Health Service.

Lerner, Gerda. 1972. *Black women in white America: A documentary history.* New York: Random House.

——. 1975. Placing women in history: A 1975 perspective. *Feminist Studies* 3, no. 102:5–15.

Levy, T. 1978. *The lesbian: As perceived by mental health workers.* Unpublished doctoral dissertation, California School of Professional Psychology, San Diego.

Liljestrand, P.; Gerling, E.; and Saliba, P. A. 1978. The effects of social sex-role stereotypes and sexual orientation on psychotherapeutic outcomes. *Journal of Homosexuality* 3, no. 4:361–372.

Lorde, Audre. 1984. *Sister outsider.* Trumansburg, N.Y.: The Crossing Press.

Luly, Margaret. 1991. Alcohol use among lesbians. Unpublished Ph.D. dissertation, University of South Carolina, Columbia.

Manley, A.; Lin-Fu, J.; Miranda, M.; Noonan, A.; and Parker, T. 1985. Special health concerns of ethnic minority women in women's health. *Report of the Public Health Service Task Force on Women's Health Issues.* Washington, D.C.: U.S. Department of Health and Human Services.

Mathews, W. C.; Booth, M. W.; Turner, J. D.; and Kessler, L. 1986. Physicians' attitudes toward homosexuality: Survey of California county medical society. *Western Journal of Medicine* 144:106–110.

McKirnan, D. J., and Peterson, P. L. 1989a. Alcohol and drug use among homosexual men and women: Epidemiology and population characteristics. *Addictive Behaviors* 14:545–553.

——. 1989b. Psychosocial and social factors in alcohol and drug abuse: An analysis of a homosexual community. *Addictive Behaviors* 14:555–563.

McNally, E. B. 1989. Lesbian recovering alcoholics in Alcoholics Anonymous: A qualitative study of identity transformation. Unpublished doctoral dissertation, School of Education, Health, Nursing, and Arts Professions, New York University.

Medical News and Perspectives. 1992. Women's Health Initiative leads way as research begins to fill gender gaps. *Journal of the American Medical Association* 267, no. 4:469–470.

Monzon, O. T., and Capellan, J. M. B. 1987. *Lancet* 2:40.

Morin, S. F. 1977. Heterosexual bias in psychological research on lesbianism and male homosexuality. *American Psychologist* 32:629–637.

Muller, Charlotte F. 1990. *Health care and gender.* New York: Russell Sage Foundation.

Multiple Risk Factor Intervention Trial Research Group. 1990. Mortality rates after 10.5 years for participants in the Multiple Risk Factor Intervention Trial: Findings related to a prior hypothesis of the trial. *Journal of the American Medicial Association* 236:1795–1801.

Norwood, Chris. 1988. Alarming rise in deaths. *Ms.* (July):65–67.

O'Donnell, M., et al. 1977. *Lesbian health matters: A resource book about lesbian health.* Santa Cruz, Calif.: Santa Cruz Women's Health Collective.

Olesker, E., and Walsh, L. V. 1984. Childbearing among lesbians: Are we meeting their needs? *Journal of Nurse-Midwifery* 29, no. 5:322–329.

Person, Ethel. 1990. The influence of values in psychoanalysis: The case of female psychology. In C. Zanardi (ed.), *Essential papers on the psychology of women,* pp. 211–267. New York: New York University Press.

Pleck, E. H. 1978. A mother's wages: Income earned among married Italian and Black women, 1896–1911. In M. Gordon (ed.), *The American family in social-historical perspective.* 2nd ed. New York: St. Martin's Press.

Radicalesbians Health Collective. 1977. Lesbians and the health care system. In K. Joy and A. Young (eds.), *Out of the closets: Voices of gay liberation,* New York: Harcourt, Brace, Jovanovich.

Randall, C. E. 1989. Lesbian phobia among BSN educators: A survey. *Journal of Nursing Education* 28:302–306.

Reagan, P. 1981. The interaction of health professionals and their lesbian clients. *Patient Counselling and Health Education* 3, no. 1:21–25.

Roberts, Joan R. 1981. *Black lesbians: An annotated bibliography.* Tallahassee, Fla.: Naiad.

Robertson, M. Morag. 1992. Lesbians as an invisible minority in the health services arena. *Health Care for Women International* 13, no. 2:155–164.

Romm, M. E. 1965. Sexuality and homosexuality in women. In J. Marmor (ed.), *Sexual inversion: The multiple roots of homosexuality,* pp. 282–301. New York: Basic Books.

Saghir, M. T., and Robins, E. 1973. *Male and female homosexuality: A comprehensive investigation.* Baltimore, Md.: The Williams and Wilkins Co.

Sahli, N. 1979. Smashing: Women's relationships before the fall. *Chrysalis* 8:17–27.

Saunders, J. M.; Tupac, J. D.; and MacCulloch, B. 1988. *A lesbian profile: A survey of 1000 lesbians.* West Hollywood, Calif.: Southern California Women for Understanding.

Schwanberg, S. L. 1985. Changes in labeling homosexuality in health sciences literature: A preliminary investigation. *Journal of Homosexuality* 12, no. 1:51–73.

———. 1990. Attitudes toward homosexuality in American health care literature 1983–1987. *Journal of Homosexuality* 19, no. 3:117–136.

Scott, Joan W. 1983. Women in history: The modern period. *Past and present: A Journal of Historical Studies* 101:141–157.

———. 1987. On language, gender, and working-class history. *International Labor and Working Class History* 31:1–13.

———. 1988. *Gender and the politics of history.* New York: Columbia University Press.

Selye, Hans. 1956. *The stress of life.* New York: McGraw-Hill Book Company.

Shilts, Randy. 1987. *And the band played on: Politics, people and the AIDS epidemic.* New York: St. Martin's Press.

Shockley, Anne. 1983. The Black lesbian in American literature. In Barbara Smith (ed.), *Home girls: A Black feminist anthology,* pp. 83–93. New York: Kitchen Table Press.

Smith, Barbara (ed.). 1983. *Home girls: A Black feminist anthology.* New York: Kitchen Table Press.

Smith, E.; Johnson, S.; and Guenther, S. 1985. Healthcare attitudes and experiences during gynecological care among lesbians and bisexuals. *American Journal of Public Health* 75:1085–1087.

Socarides, C. W. 1968. *The overt homosexual.* New York: Grune and Stratton.

Staples, Ruth. 1973. *The Black woman in America.* Chicago: Nelson-Hall Co.

Steering Committee of the Physician's Health Study Group. 1989. Final report on the aspirin component of the ongoing physician's health study. *New England Journal of Medicine* 321:129–135.

Stevens, Patricia E. 1992. Lesbian health care research: A review of the literature from 1970 to 1990. *Health Care for Women International* 13, no. 2:91–120.

Stevens, P. E., and Hall, J. M. 1988. Stigma, health beliefs, and experiences with health care in lesbian women. *Image: Journal of Nursing Scholarship* 10, no. 2:69–73.

———. 1990. Abusive health care interactions experienced by lesbians: A case of institutional violence in the treatment of women. *Response: To the victimization of women and children* 13, no. 3:23–27.

Swanson, D. W.; Loomis, S. D.; Lukesh, R. C.; Cronin, R.; and Smith, J. A. 1972. Clinical features of the female homosexual patient. *The Journal of Nervous and Mental Disease* 155, no. 2:119–124.

Tallen, Bette S. 1990. Twelve step programs: A lesbian feminist critique. *NWSA Journal* 2, no. 3:390–407.

Thompson, C. 1950. Some effects of the derogatory attitude towards female sexuality. *Psychiatry* 13:349–354.

Trippet, Susan E., and Joyce Bain. 1992. Reasons American lesbians fail to seek traditional health care. *Health Care for Women International* 13, no. 2:145–154.

Turbin, C. 1979. And we are nothing but women: Irish working women in Troy. In C. R. Berkin and M. B. Norton (eds.), *Women of America: A history*. Boston: Houghton Mifflin.

Underhill, B. L., and Ostermann, S. E. 1991. The pain of invisibility: Issues for lesbians. In P. Roth (ed.), *Alcohol and drugs are women's issues*, vol. 1: *A review of the issues*. Metuchen, N.J.: Women's Action Alliance and the Scarecrow Press.

Watters, A. T. 1986. Heterosexual bias in psychological research on lesbianism and male homosexuality (1979–1983): Utilizing the bibliographic and taxonomic system of Morin (1977). *Journal of Homosexuality* 13, no. 1:35–58.

Weathers, B. 1981. *Alcoholism and the lesbian community*. Washington, D.C.: Gay Council on Drinking Behavior.

West, C. 1987. Lesbian daughter. *Sage: A Scholarly Journal on Black Women* 4, no. 2:42–44.

White, Deborah. 1991. The cost of club work, the price of black feminism. In S. Lebsock and N. Hewitt (eds.), *Invincible women*. Urbana: University of Illinois Press.

White, T. A. 1979. Attitudes of psychiatric nurses toward same sex orientations. *Nursing Research* 28, no. 5:276–281.

Wilbur, C. B. 1965. Clinical aspects of female homosexuality. In J. Marmor (ed.), *Sexual inversion: The multiple roots of homosexuality*, pp. 268–281. New York: Basic Books.

Wolff, C. 1971. *Love between women*. New York: Harper and Row.

Young, E. W. 1988. Nurses' attitudes toward homosexuality: Analysis of change in AIDS workshops. *Journal of Continuing Education in Nursing* 19, no. 1:9–12.

Young, I. 1981. Beyond the unhappy marriage: A critique of the dual systems theory. In L. Sargent (ed.), *Women and revolution: A discussion of the unhappy marriage of Marxism and feminism*. Boston: South End Press.

Zeidenstein, L. 1990. Gynecological and childbearing needs of lesbians. *Journal of Nurse-Midwifery* 35, no. 1:10–18.

Part Three

INCLUDING WOMEN IN
MEDICAL EDUCATION

CHAPTER EIGHT

Feminist Methodologies and Clinical Research

The politics of health care and health care reform serve as the focus of considerable current debate as the Clinton administration seeks to solve the national health care crisis. With Hillary Rodham Clinton as chair of the committee on health reform, Donna Shalala as secretary of Health and Human Services, and the newly instituted changes at the National Institutes of Health (NIH), including the Office for Research on Women and the Women's Health Initiative, women's health has begun to move from the margins toward the center of the discussion. Feminists have been invited and encouraged to participate in the multiple meetings such as the 40th Annual National Health Forum on Health for Women in the 21st Century and the First Annual Congress on Women's Health held in Washington, D.C., during June 1993.

Large numbers of feminists are involved in various aspects of health care reform, ranging from policy formation through access and delivery. A considerable body of research evolved by women's studies scholars working through the traditional disciplines such as political science, public health, nursing, and social work provides feminist frameworks through which to suggest and evaluate proposed reforms. Sufficient numbers of scholars representing a variety of theoretical perspectives, including liberal, socialist, African-American, and radical feminist, exist to provide some insights into possible advantages and disadvantages of various changes from the standpoints of different groups of women.

Policy formation, widening access, and improving delivery represent crucial issues which must be resolved in order to improve health care in the United States. It is particularly important that feminist perspectives be voiced on those issues as changes are made. Basic scientific and clinical research constitutes an equally significant area for health care reform. Often the priorities for research, the topics chosen for study, the subpopulations of individuals included in and excluded from research protocols, and the theories and conclusions drawn from the data set the parameters for policy, access, and delivery. Women and feminist voices have been largely absent from the discussions of research agendas.

The full range of women's voices is needed now more than ever to consider potential impacts of proposed health care reforms. Feminist voices representing a variety of political positions and theoretical perspectives must scrutinize the research, including the clinical studies upon which the reforms are based. When bias in choice of topics for study and exclusion of women from research protocols enters at the stage of research design, it may be translated into distortions and absences for each step of health care, ultimately resulting in poorer treatment and increased death rates for women.

An exploration of the differing methodologies appropriate for clinical research derived from various feminist theories may help in the evaluation of research designs and approaches. Examination of the questions raised about feminist methodologies for sciences and clinical research reveals that the answers are complex and dependent upon the feminist theory from which the methodology springs. The jumble of descriptors for feminist methodology—rejects dualisms, is based on women's experience, shortens the distance between observer and object of study, rejects unicausal, hierarchical approaches, unites application with problem—seem like an unlikely conglomerate when portrayed as feminist methodology. They become much more understandable when viewed as a lumping together of possible methodological implications for science resulting from different feminist theories.

FEMINIST THEORIES

Individuals unfamiliar with feminism or women's studies might assume that feminist theory provides a singular and unified framework for analysis. In one sense this is correct; all feminist theory posits gender as a significant characteristic that interacts with other factors such as race and class to structure relationships between individuals, within groups, and within society as a whole. However, viewing the world through the lens of gender results in diverse images or theories: liberal feminism, Marxist feminism, socialist feminism, African-American feminism, lesbian separatist feminism, conservative or essentialist feminism, existential feminism, psychoanalytic feminism, and radical feminism. The variety and complexity of these various theories provide a framework through which to explore interesting issues of methodology raised in clinical research.

LIBERAL FEMINISM

Since the eighteenth century, political scientists, philosophers, and feminists (Wollstonecraft, 1975; J. S. Mill, 1970; H. T. Mill, 1970; Friedan, 1974; Jaggar, 1983) have described the parameters of liberal feminism. Nineteenth- and twentieth-century liberal feminists have ranged from libertarian to egalitarian, and numerous complexities exist among definitions of liberal feminists today. However, a general definition of liberal feminism is the belief that women are suppressed in contemporary society because they suffer unjust discrimination (Jaggar, 1983). Liberal feminists seek no special privileges for women and simply demand that everyone receive equal consideration without discrimination on the basis of sex.

Most scientists would assume that the implications of liberal feminism for medicine and clinical research are that scientists should work to remove the documented overt and covert barriers (National Science Foundation, 1990; Rosser, 1990; Vetter, 1988; Rossiter, 1982) that have prevented women from entering and succeeding in science. Although they might hold individual opinions as to whether women deserve equal pay for equal work, equal access to research resources, and equal opportunities for advancement, most scientists, even those who are brave enough to call themselves feminists, assume that the implications of liberal feminism extend only to employment, access, and discrimination issues.

In fact, its implications extend beyond this. Liberal feminism shares two fundamental assumptions with the foundations of the traditional method for scientific discovery: (1) both assume that human beings are highly individualistic and obtain knowledge in a rational manner that may be separated from their social conditions, and (2) both accept positivism as the theory of knowledge. Positivism implies that "all knowledge is constructed by inference from immediate sensory experiences" (Jaggar, 1983, pp. 355–356). These two assumptions lead to a belief in the possibilities of obtaining knowledge that is both objective and value-free, concepts which form the cornerstone of the scientific method. The notion of objectivity involves the assumption that similar sensory experiences or circumstances would stimulate similar perceptions in individuals with normal faculties of perception even when those perceptions occur at different times or places to the separate individuals. In order for these sensations to be perceived in the same way, the individuals must rely only upon their empirical observations and control their own values, interests, and emotions. Objectivity is thus contingent upon value neutrality or freedom from values, interests, and emotions associated with a particular class, race, or sex. Double-blind studies and quantitative approaches represent attempts at objective methodologies which are frequently used in clinical research.

Although each scientist strives to be as objective and value-free as possible, most scientists, feminists, and philosophers of science recognize that no individual can be completely neutral. Instead "objectivity is defined to mean independence from the value judgments of any particular individual" (Jaggar, 1983, p. 357).

In the past two decades, feminist historians and philosophers of science (Fee, 1982; Harding, 1986; Haraway, 1990) and feminist scientists (Bleier, 1984, 1986; Fausto-Sterling, 1985; Birke, 1986; Keller, 1983, 1985; Rosser, 1988; Spanier, 1982) have pointed out a source of bias and absence of value neutrality in science, particularly biology. Through the exclusion of females as experimental subjects, a focus on problems of primary interest to males, faulty experimental designs, and interpretations of data based in language or ideas constricted by patriarchal parameters, experimental results in several areas in biology have been demonstrated to be biased or flawed. Feminist critiques (Keller, 1985; Harding, 1986) suggest that these flaws and biases were permitted to become part of the mainstream of scientific thought and were perpetuated in the scientific literature for decades, in some cases (Sayers, 1982) for more than a century, because virtually all scientists were men. Therefore values held by most males were not distinguishable as biasing; they became synonymous with the "objective" view of the world.

Two examples illustrate the flawed research resulting from male bias in clinical research:

Male Animal and Human Models

Some researchers have observed behavior in lower animals in a search for "universal" behavior patterns that occur in males of all species or in all males of a particular order or class such as primates or mammals. This behavior is then extrapolated to humans in an attempt to demonstrate a biological or innate basis for the behavior.

Feminist critiques have centered on the assumption that behaviors such as aggression, homosexuality, promiscuity, selfishness, and altruism are biologically determined. Problems involving anthropomorphism in animal behavior studies are also underlined. The anthropomorphism occurs in at least two forms: (a) the use of human language and frameworks to describe animal behavior which is then used to "prove" that certain human behaviors are innate since they are also found in animals, and (b) the selective choice of species for study that mirror human society.

Although it was clear in the early primatology work (Yerkes, 1943) that particular primate species, such as the baboon and chimpanzee, were chosen for study primarily because their social organization was seen by observers as closely resembling that of human primates, subsequent researchers forgot the "obvious" limitations imposed by such selection of species and proceeded to generalize the data to universal behavior patterns for all primates. It was not until a significant number of women entered primatology that concepts of the universality and male leadership of dominance hierarchies among primates (Lancaster, 1975; Leavitt, 1975; Leibowitz, 1975; Rowell, 1974) were questioned and shown to be inaccurate for many primate species. The "evident" problems discussed by feminist critics (Bleier, 1984) of studying nonhuman primates in an attempt to discover what the true nature of humans would be without the overlay of culture, have also been largely ignored by many of the sociobiologists and scientists studying animal behavior.

The favored methodology for experimental testing of drugs employs the double-blind study. In a double-blind study, neither the researcher nor the subjects know who among the subjects receives the true drug and who receives the placebo. This method is thought to ensure objectivity, since neither party is biased by knowing who receives the drug.

Feminists have revealed a source of bias in many double-blind studies which were run using only male rats, human beings, or other primates as experimental subjects. Perhaps the notion that the double-blind study ensures objectivity made the researchers overly confident of their results. In many cases (Steering Committee of the Physician's Health Study Group, 1989; U.S. GAO, 1990), researchers universalized the results beyond what the data warranted to the entire population. Because the studies were done on males only and because the differing levels of hormones in males and females frequently cause significantly different interactions with drugs in the two sexes, this extrapolation from the study population of males only to the entire human species is inaccurate and inappropriate.

Sex Differences Research

In the neurosciences, a substantial amount of work has been done relating to sex differences in the brains of men and women. Studies on brain lateralization, genes, brain structure, and effects of prenatal and postpubertal androgens and estrogens on the nervous system have been carried out in an attempt to discern biological bases for differences between males and females in behavioral or performance characteristics such as aggression or verbal, visuo-spatial, and mathematical ability. Excellent critiques have been made by feminists of the faulty experimental designs and unfounded extrapolations beyond the data of the work in brain lateralization (Star, 1979), hormones (Bleier, 1984), genes (Fennema and Sherman, 1977), and brain structure (Bleier, 1986). Although most scientists accept the validity of the critiques, reputable scientific journals (see Bleier, 1988, for an account of her encounters with *Science* over this matter), textbooks, and the popular press continue to publish studies biased by similar methodological inconsistencies, extrapolations of data from one species to another, and overgeneralizations of data.

These examples of flawed research and other examples resulting from the critiques of feminists have raised fundamental questions regarding gender and good science: Do these examples simply represent "bad science"? Is good science really gender-free, or does the scientific method when properly used permit research that is objective and unbiased?

The liberal feminist answer to these questions is that good science can be gender-free. Liberal feminists (Keller, 1984) suggest that now that the bias of gender has been revealed by the feminist critique, scientists can take it into account and correct for it. A liberal feminist position has two significant implications:

1. It does not question the integrity of the scientific method itself or of its supporting corollaries of objectivity and value neutrality. Liberal

feminism reaffirms the idea that it is possible to find a perspective from which to observe that is truly impartial, rational, and detached. Liberal feminism would accept the double-blind study. Lack of objectivity and the presence of bias occur because of human failure to properly follow the scientific method and avoid bias due to a situation or condition such as inappropriate extrapolation beyond what the data warrant (for example, from only male experimental subjects to the entire human population) in a double-blind study. Liberal feminists argue that it was through attempts to become more value-neutral that the possible androcentrism in previous scientific research was revealed.

2. Liberal feminism also implies that good scientific research is not conducted differently by men and women, and that in principle men can be just as good feminists as women. Now that feminist critiques have revealed flaws in research due to gender bias, both men and women will use this revelation to design experiments which include both male and female subjects, gather and interpret data, and draw conclusions and theories that are more objective and free from bias, including gender bias (Biology and Gender Study Group, 1989).

In contrast to liberal feminism, all other feminist theories call into question the fundamental assumptions underlying the scientific method, its corollaries of objectivity and value neutrality, or its implications. They reject individualism for a social construction of knowledge and question positivism and the possibility of obtaining objectivity by value neutrality. Many also imply that men and women may conduct scientific research differently, although each theory posits a different cause for the gender distinction. Just as examination of liberal feminism uncovered interesting information about methodology in clinical research, exploration of other feminist theories reveals fruitful points.

MARXIST FEMINISM

Marxist feminism contrasts with liberal feminism in its rejection of individualism and positivism as approaches to knowledge. Marxist critiques of science, the historical precursors of Marxist feminist critiques, view all knowledge as socially constructed and originating from practical human involvement in production that takes a definite historic form. According to Marxism, knowledge, including scientific knowledge, cannot be solely individualistic. Since knowledge is a productive activity of human beings, it cannot be objective and value-free because its basic categories are shaped by human purposes and values. Marxism proposes that the form of knowledge is determined by the prevailing mode of production. In the twentieth-century United States, according to Marxism, scientific knowledge would be determined by capitalism and reflect the interests of the dominant class. In strict Marxist feminism, where class is emphasized over gender, only bourgeois (liberal) feminism or proletarian feminism can exist. The research produced by a bourgeois woman researcher would be expected to be the same as that produced by a bourgeois man researcher but different from that produced by a proletarian woman researcher.

Although feminists have criticized Marxism for decades (Goldman, 1931; Foreman, 1977; Vogel, 1983; Flax, 1981) about its shortcomings on the woman question, the Marxist critique of science opened the door to three insights shared by feminist theories and methodologies:

1. It proposed that scientific knowledge was socially constructed and could not be dichotomized from other human values the scientist holds. Beginning with the work of Thomas Kuhn (1970) and his followers, historians and philosophers of science have pointed out that the scientific paradigms that are acceptable to the mainstream of practicing scientists are convincing precisely because they reinforce or support the historical, economic, and social, racial, political, and gender policies of the majority of scientists at that particular time.

The use of craniometry in the nineteenth century provides an example. Incorrect biological measurements and false conclusions drawn from accurate measurements were accepted because the biological "facts" provided a justification for the inferior social position of colonials (especially Blacks) and women (Gould, 1981).

Feminist critics (Bleier, 1984, 1986; Fee, 1982; Haraway, 1978; Hein, 1981; Hubbard, 1979) have discussed the extent to which the emphasis upon sex differences research (when in fact for most traits there are no differences or only very small mean differences characterized by a large range of overlap between the sexes) in the neurosciences and endocrinology and upon the search for genetic bases to justify sex role specialization and the division of labor originate from the desire to find a biological basis for the social inequality between the sexes. The measurement of hormone levels in homosexuals compared to heterosexuals, the search for anatomical differences between the brains of homosexuals and heterosexuals, and the search for a "gene" for homosexuality are an attempt to separate biological from environmental determinants and to seek biological bases for the discriminatory treatment against homosexuals (Birke, 1986). One can imagine that a society free from inequality between the sexes and lacking homophobia would not view sex differences and sexual preferences differences research as valid scientific endeavors. The fact that our society supports such research indicates the extent to which the values of the society and the scientists influence scientific inequity and "objectivity."

2. By emphasizing the social construction of knowledge, Marxism implies that dichotomies such as nature/culture, subjective/objective might not be the only or even appropriate ways to categorize knowledge. Interdisciplinary methods which study disease processes such as cardiovascular disease, cancer, and menopause based on interactions between genetic and environmental factors would be more in tune with Marxist approaches.

3. It also suggests that methods which distance the observer from the object of study and/or place the experimenter in a different plane from the subject are seen as more scientific only when the social construction of knowledge is not recognized.

The privileging of double-blind studies and quantitative methods may no longer seem as valid when knowledge is acknowledged to be socially constructed. Active participation of subjects in research and qualitative methods may then be viewed as a superior way to study health problems. Elizabeth Fee outlines the advantages to such an approach using the example of occupational health research in an Italian factory:

> Prior to 1969, occupational health research was done by specialists who would be asked by management to investigate a potential problem in the factory. . . . The procedure was rigorously objective, the results were submitted to management. The workers were the individualized and passive objects of this kind of research. In 1969, however, when workers' committees were established in the factories, they refused to allow this type of investigation. . . . Occupational health specialists had to discuss the ideas and procedures of research with workers' assemblies and see their "objective" expertise measured against the "subjective" experience of the workers. The mutual validation of data took place by testing in terms of the workers' experience of reality and not simply by statistical methods; the subjectivity of the workers' experience was involved at each level in the definition of the problem, the method of research, and the evaluation of solutions. Their collective experience was understood to be much more than the statistical combination of individual data; the workers had become the active subjects of research, involved in the production, evaluation, and uses of the knowledge relating to their own experience. (Fee, 1983, p. 24)

AFRICAN-AMERICAN CRITIQUE

African-American or Black feminism also rejects individualism and positivism in favor of social construction as an approach to knowledge. In addition to repudiating the objectivity and value neutrality associated with the positivist approach accepted by liberal feminism, the African-American approach critiques dichotomization of knowledge, or at least the identification of science with the first half and African-American with the latter half of the following dichotomies: culture/nature; rational/feeling; objective/subjective; quantitative/qualitative; active/passive; focused/diffuse; independent/dependent; mind/body; self/others; knowing/being (Harding, 1986). Like Marxism, African-American critiques question methods that distance the observer from the object of study, thereby denying a facet of the social construction of knowledge.

Whereas Marxism posits class as the organizing principle around which the struggle for power exists, African-American critiques maintain that race is the primary cause of oppression. Neo-Marxists view the entire scientific and health care enterprise as a function of context and class-specific interests, with methodology itself constituted by these interests. African-Americans critical of these enterprises may see them as a function of white Eurocentric interests. The Tuskegee syphilis experiments studied the effects of untreated syphilis in 399 African-American men over a period of forty years (Jones, 1981). The failure of the white middle-class researchers to see the "flaw" in allowing these poor African-American men to go untreated when a cure for syphilis was known demonstrates both race and class interests in research methodology. Just as Marxists view class oppression as primary and superseding gender oppression, African-American critiques place race oppression above that of gender. A strict, traditional interpretation would suggest that research produced by African-American women would more closely resemble research produced by African-American men than that produced by white women.

Many feminists were attracted by certain tenets—particularly the ideas of the social construction of knowledge, rejection of objectivity and other dualisms, and locating the observer in the same plane as the object of study—of both Marxist and African-American critiques. However, as feminists they had experienced and recognized the oppression of gender and found it unacceptable to have it ignored or subsumed as a secondary oppression under class or race. Both socialist feminism and African-American feminism have examined the respective intersection of class and gender or race and gender in an attempt to provide a more complex and comprehensive view of reality.

SOCIALIST FEMINISM AND AFRICAN-AMERICAN FEMINISM

The addition of socialist feminism and African-American feminism to classical Marxist and African-American critiques is based on the assertion that the special position of women within (or as) a class or race gives them a special standpoint that provides them with a particular world view. This female world view is supposedly more reliable and less distorted than that of men from the same class or race. Implicit in the acceptance of the social construction of knowledge is the rejection of the neutral, disinterested observer of liberal feminism. Marxist and African-American critiques suggest that the prevailing knowledge and science reflect the interests and values of the dominant race and class. Because the dominant race and class have an interest in concealing, and may not in fact recognize, the way they dominate, the research and picture of reality they present will be distorted.

In contemporary health care research, for example, the identification of AIDS by group characteristics such as sexual orientation, class, and race—gay males, IV drug users, and Haitian immigrants—rather than risk behaviors demonstrates the ability of the dominant heterosexual, white middle class to label the disease as "other" and distort the research agenda. The intensive study of crack-cocaine and other substance abuse in women (primarily poor and African-American) seeking prenatal care in public health settings coupled with the lack of study of such abuse in women obtaining prenatal care in private-practice settings demonstrates similar dominance and distortion (Chasnoff, Landress, and Barrett, 1990).

Classical Marxist and African-American critiques suggest that individuals oppressed by class and/or race have an advantageous and more comprehensive view of reality. Because of their oppression, they have an interest in perceiving problems with the status quo and the science, knowledge, and health care research produced by the dominant class and race. Simultaneously, their position requires them to understand the science and condition of the dominant group in order to survive. Thus, the standpoint of the oppressed comprehends and includes that of the dominant group, so it is superior.

Socialist feminist (Jaggar, 1983; Hartmann, 1981; Mitchell, 1971, 1974; Young, 1980, 1981) and African-American feminist critiques assert that in contemporary society, women suffer oppression because of their gender. Women oppressed by both class and gender (socialist feminists) or both race and gender (African-American feminists) have a more comprehensive, inclusive standpoint than do working-class men or Black men. Socialist feminist and African-American feminist theory imply that women scientists, through a collective process of political and scientific struggle (Jaggar, 1983), might produce a science and knowledge different from that produced by men of any race or class.

This research would provide a more accurate picture of reality since it would be based in the experience of women, who hold a more comprehensive view because of their race, class, and gender. The National Black Women's Health Project, founded by Byllye Avery, exemplifies this view in its attempts to define health care issues and education from the standpoint of African-American women.

Other feminist theories also maintain that women, because they are women, possess a different perspective or standpoint than men. Common to these theories is the assumption that diversity among women due to race, class, religion, ethnic background, sexual orientation, age, and other factors exists. However, gender is a predominant factor which provides women with a sufficiently unique and unified perspective that their knowledge, science, and view of reality are likely to differ from that of men. The primary difference among these other feminist theories is their position on the source of gender differences between men and women. Thus some variation exists among them about its effects upon methodology.

ESSENTIALIST FEMINISM

Essentialist feminism posits that women are different from men because of their biology, specifically their secondary sex characteristics and their reproductive systems. Frequently this theory may be extended to include gender differences in visuo-spatial and verbal ability, aggression and other behavior, and other physical and mental traits based on prenatal or pubertal hormone exposure. Nineteenth-century essentialist feminists (Blackwell, [1885] 1976; Calkins, 1896; Tanner, 1896) often accepted the ideas of male essentialist scientists such as Freud ("anatomy is destiny" [1924]) or Darwin, as interpreted by the social Darwinists, that there are innate differences between men and women. These early feminists proposed that the biologically based gender differences meant that women were inferior to men in some physical (Blackwell, 1976; Smith-Rosenberg, 1975) and mental (Tanner, 1896; Hollingsworth, 1914) traits, but that they were superior in others. Biological essentialism formed the basis for the supposed moral superiority of women which nineteenth-century suffragettes (DuBois et al., 1985; Hartmann and Banner, 1974) used as a persuasive argument for giving women the vote.

In the earlier phases of the current wave of feminism, most feminist scientists (Bleier, 1979; Hubbard, 1979; Rosser, 1982; Fausto-Sterling, 1985) fought against some sociobiological research such as that by Wilson (1975), Trivers (1972), and Dawkins (1976) and some hormone and brain lateralization research (Gorski et al., 1980; Goy and Phoenix, 1971; Sperry, 1974; Buffery and Gray, 1972) which seemed to provide biological evidence for differences in mental and behavioral characteristics between males and females. Essentialism was seen as a tool for conservatives who wished to keep women in the home and out of the workplace. More recently, feminists have reexamined essentialism from perspectives ranging from conservative (Fox-Genovese, 1991) to radical (MacKinnon, 1982, 1987; Corea, 1985; Rich, 1976; Dworkin, 1983; O'Brien, 1981), with a recognition that biologically based differences between the sexes might imply superiority and power for women in some arenas.

Essentialist feminism would imply that because of their biology, differential hormonal effects on the brain, the physical experiences of menstrual cycles, pregnancy, childbirth, lactation, and menopause, and/or other differing anatomical or physiological characteristics, women researchers would produce a different science from that of men. It seems logical and understandable that as a result of their biological experiences women might be interested in different problems than men. However, essentialism would imply that these differences would lead them to different methods in approaching these problems; i.e., experiencing menstruation might lead women to different methods from those used by men for studying menstruation.

Some of the differences described by scholars (Ehrenreich and English, 1978; Sullivan and Weitz, 1988; Arnup, Levesque, and Pierson, 1990; Wertz and Wertz, 1977) between the way that female midwives and male physicians solve difficulties arising during labor and childbirth might be perceived as essentialist. For example, the emphasis of midwives on emotional and spiritual support for the laboring mother while taking time to massage the perineum during the emergence of the baby's head might be construed as arising from the remembrance by the midwife of how her own body felt during labor and childbirth. In contrast, the male physician, having never personally undergone labor or childbirth, favors drugs to deaden the pain and surgical procedures such as episiotomies to speed the delivery, thereby shortening the ordeal.

A contradiction within essentialist feminism would seem to be that although it rejects the positivist "neutral observer" standpoint of liberal feminism, its relationship with the social construction of knowledge seems somewhat different from that of other feminist theories. Liberal feminism is usually equated not only with the positivist neutral observer but also with nonessentialism, or at least the assumption of equality between the sexes. Essentialism is based on biological differences between men and women rather than the social construction of gender posited by other feminist theories, including liberal feminism. Yet essentialist feminism, in its suggestion that male and female researchers might approach problems differently because of their gender, implies a social construction of knowledge and clinical research.

EXISTENTIALIST FEMINISM

Existentialist feminism, first described by Simone de Beauvoir (1974), suggests that women's "otherness" and the social construction of gender rest on society's interpretation of biological differences:

> The enslavement of the female to the species and the limitations of her various powers are extremely important facts; the body of woman is one of the essential elements in her situation in the world. But that body is not enough to define her as woman; there is no true living reality except as manifested by the conscious individual through activities and in the bosom of a society. Biology is not enough to give an answer to the question that is before us: why is woman the Other? (P. 51)

In other words, it is the value that society assigns to biological differences between males and females which has led women to play the role of the Other (Tong, 1989); it is not the biological differences themselves. It is possible to imagine a society without gender differences.

The methodological implications arising out of existentialist feminism are that a society which emphasizes gender differences would produce a science which emphasizes sex differences. In such a society, men and women might be expected to create very different sciences because of the social construction of both gender and science. The possibility of a gender-free or gender-neutral (positivist) science evolving in such a society is virtually nil. Elizabeth Fee summed up the situation very well: she states that a sexist society should be expected to develop a sexist science. Conceptualizing a feminist science from within our society is "like asking a medieval peasant to imagine the theory of genetics or the production of a space capsule" (1982, p. 31).

Existentialist feminism provides a theoretical explanation for the current significant gender differential in research and treatment in cardiovascular disease in men compared to women. Because this society defines women as "other" in contrast to men, the fact that heart disease strikes men at an earlier age than women served as sufficient reason to direct the vast majority of research funds and treatment protocols toward men. The similar frequency of heart disease in women compared to men was ignored since difference in age rather than similarity of frequency was emphasized in keeping with the definition of women as "other." This emphasis on difference resulted in extreme bias in research, such as women's exclusion from 82 percent of studies of clinical trials between 1960 and 1991 for medications to prevent myocardial infarctions (Gurwitz, Nananda, and Avorn, 1992) and an in-hospital death rate for women ten times that of men after angioplasty (Kelsey et al., 1993).

PSYCHOANALYTIC FEMINISM

In many ways, psychoanalytic feminism takes a stance similar to that of existentialist feminism. Derived from Freudian theory, psychoanalysis posits that girls and boys develop contrasting gender roles because they experience their sexuality differently and deal differently with the stages of psychosexual development. Based on the Freudian prejudice that anatomy is destiny, psychoanalytic theory assumes that biological sex will lead to different ways for boys and girls to resolve the Oedipus and castration complexes which arise during the phallic stage of normal sexual development. As was the situation with existentialism, psychoanalysis recognizes that gender construction is not biologically essential; in "normal" gender construction the biological sex of the child-caretaker interaction differs depending on the sex of the child (and possibly that of the primary caretaker). However, psychoanalytic theory is not strictly biologically deterministic, since cases of "abnormal" sexuality may result when gender construction is opposite to or not congruent with biological sex.

Simone de Beauvoir admired Freud for advancing the idea that sexuality is the ultimate explanation for the form of civilization and gender relations (Tong, 1989). However, she criticized Freud's interpretation as overly simplistic. She particularly rejected his theory of women's castration complex as a psychological explanation for their inferior social status. De Beauvoir suggested that the reason women may suffer from so-called penis envy is that they desire the material and psychological privileges permitted men in our society rather than the anatomical organ itself.

Numerous feminists (Firestone, 1970; Friedan, 1974; Millett, 1970) in the 1960s and 1970s attacked Freud and the successor psychoanalytic theories because of their negative view of women and the considerable damage that application of those theories had done to women's sexuality. They also read his statement "anatomy is destiny" as a major impediment to reforms allowing women to work outside the home and to assume other prominent roles in public life. Changes in social structures will not change gender relationships if the root of the problem is biological rather than social.

In recent years, a number of feminists have again become interested in Freud's theories. Rejecting the biological determinism in Freud, Dinnerstein (1977) and Chodorow (1978) in particular have used an aspect of psychoanalytic theory known as object-relations theory to look at the construction of gender and sexuality. Chodorow and Dinnerstein examine the Oedipal stage of psychosexual development to determine why the construction of gender and sexuality in this stage usually results in male dominance. They conclude that the gender differences resulting in male dominance can be traced to the fact that in our society, women are the primary caretakers for most infants and children.

Accepting most Freudian ideas about the Oedipus complex, Chodorow and Dinnerstein conclude that boys are pushed to be independent, distant, and autonomous from their female caretakers while girls are permitted to be more dependent, intimate, and less individuated from their mothers or female caretakers. Building upon the work of Chodorow and Dinnerstein, feminists (Keller, 1982; Harding, 1986; Hein, 1981) have explored how the gender identity proposed by object-relations theory with women as caretakers might lead to more men choosing careers in science. Keller (1982, 1985) in particular applied the work of Chodorow and Dinnerstein to suggest how science has become a masculine province which excludes women and causes them to exclude themselves from it. Science is a masculine province not only in the fact that it is populated mostly by men but also in the choice of experimental topics, the use of male subjects for experimentation, interpretation of and theorizing from data, as well as the practice and applications of science undertaken by the scientists. Keller suggests (1982, 1985) that since the scientific method stresses objectivity, rationality, distance, and autonomy of the observer from the object of study (i.e., the positivist neutral observer), individuals who feel comfortable with independence, autonomy, and distance will be most likely to become scientists. Because most caretakers during the Oedipal phase are female, most of the individuals in our culture who will be comfortable as scientists will be male. The type of science they create will also be reflective of those same characteristics of independence, distance, and autonomy. It is on this basis that feminists have suggested that the objectivity and rationality of science are synonymous with a male approach to the physical, natural world.

Keller's theory is compatible with the data demonstrating that many more male than female physicians pursue careers in clinical research. For example, only one-sixteenth of the faculty in U.S. medical schools holding M.D.–Ph.D. degrees are female (Sherman, Johnson, and Whiting, 1990, p. 31). Since the proportion of women students in medical school approaches 40 percent (Section for Student Services, 1992), one would anticipate that more than 6.5 percent of M.D.–Ph.D. faculty would be women. Similarly, 34.6 percent (4,627 out of 13,359) of women medical school faculty are on non-tenure track, compared to 25.8 percent (13,334 out of 51,647) of men faculty. (Data calculated from Sherman, Johnson, and Whiting, 1990, tables IIA and B, pp. 25–26.) Factors such as correspondence between the biological time clock for childbearing, financial burdens of pursuing extended education such as Ph.D. and M.D. programs, and social expectations that women take primary responsibility for child care provide more obvious pragmatic explanations than psychoanalytic feminism for why fewer women undertake research in clinical medicine than men. However, these factors reinforce the notion of women as primary caretakers, which serves as the basis for the origin of gender difference under psychoanalytic feminism.

According to psychoanalytic feminism, women researchers might be more likely to use approaches that shorten the distance between them as observer and their object of study, might develop a relationship with their object of study, and might appear to be less objective. The biography of Barbara McClintock, *A Feeling for the Organism,* written by Evelyn Fox Keller (1983), demonstrates this. McClintock's statement on receiving the Nobel Prize was that "it might seem unfair to reward a person for having so much pleasure over the years, asking the maize plant to solve specific problems and then watching its responses" (Keller, 1983). Works by Goodfield (1981) and Hynes (1989) have also discussed this more "feminine" approach taken by women researchers.

Comparisons of approaches to clinical research undertaken by nurses and physicians reveal that nurses favor qualitative, patient-involved approaches, while physicians favor quantitative, double-blind studies. Complex social, economic, and gender interactions have resulted in the female-dominated profession of nursing, emphasizing caring, qualitative, patient-centered, and involved research, and the male-dominated medical profession using "objective," quantitative research where distance is maintained between the patient and the physician researcher. Numerous scholars have explored these interactions in depth and have revealed their complexities. Although psychoanalytic feminism may oversimplify these historical, economic, class, and gender complexities, it is compatible with the differential research approaches of nursing and medicine.

Psychoanalytic feminism does not necessarily imply that biological males will take a masculine approach and that biological females will take a feminine approach. In most cases, as a result of the resolution of the Oedipal complex with a female caretaker, this will be the case. Proponents of psychoanalytic feminism (Keller, 1985) suggest that this is why so many more males than females are attracted to science. However, many of the biological females who are currently researchers probably take a more masculine approach, a result not only of resolution of psychosexual development phases but also of training by male scientists and physicians. Psychoanalytic feminism also suggests that biological males could take a "feminine" approach.

Psychoanalytic feminism also opens the door to "gender-neutral" or "gender-free" (Keller, 1984) science. Chodorow (1978) and Dinnerstein (1977) find that the solution to gender differences which result in male dominance is having the father or another male take a much more active role in caring for the child. They suggest that the active involvement of both women and men in caretaking will lead children to recognize that both men and women have strengths and weaknesses. It would also presumably result in less polarization in gender roles and the possibility of a gender-free science. Although the gender-free potential of psychoanalytic feminism seems similar to the neutral, detached observer of liberal feminism, psychoanalytic feminism is premised on a type of social construction of knowledge—knowledge of sexuality and gender.

RADICAL FEMINISM

Radical feminism, in contrast to psychoanalytic and liberal feminism, rejects the possibility of gender-free research or a science developed from a neutral, objective perspective. Radical feminism maintains that women's oppression is the first, most widespread, and deepest oppression (Jaggar and Rothenberg, 1984). Since men dominate and control most institutions, politics, and knowledge in our society, they reflect a male perspective and are effective in oppressing women. Scientific and medical institutions, practice, and knowledge are particularly male-dominated and have been documented by many feminists (Merchant, 1979; Griffin, 1978; Fee, 1982; Haraway, 1978, 1990; Rosser, 1990; Bleier, 1984; Hubbard, 1990; Keller, 1985) to be especially effective patriarchal tools for controlling and harming women. Radical feminism rejects most scientific and medical theories, data, and experiments not only because they exclude women but also because they are not women-centered.

The theory that radical feminism proposes is evolving (Tong, 1989). Its theory is less developed than some of the other feminist theories discussed above for reasons that spring fairly directly from the nature of radical feminism itself. First, it is radical. That means that it rejects most of the currently accepted ideas about scientific epistemology—what kinds of things can be known, who can be a knower, and how beliefs are legitimated as knowledge—and methodology—the general structure of how theory finds its application in particular scientific disciplines. Second, unlike the feminisms previously discussed, radical feminism does not have its basis in a theory such as Marxism, positivism, psychoanalysis, or existentialism, already developed for decades by men. Since radical feminism is based in women's experience, it rejects feminisms rooted in theories developed by men based on their experience and world view. Third, the theory of radical feminism must be developed by women and based in women's experience (MacKinnon, 1987). Because radical feminism maintains that the oppression of women is the deepest, most widespread, and historically first oppression, women have had few opportunities to come together, understand their experiences collectively, and develop theories based on those experiences.

Not surprisingly, the implications of radical feminism for science and medicine and the scientific method and medical research are much more far-reaching than those of other feminist theories. Radical feminism implies rejection of much of the standard epistemology of science. It perceives reality as an inseparable whole, always alive and in motion, both spiritual and material (Capra, 1973), so that connections between humans and other parts of the natural and physical world constitute part of what can be known (Jaggar, 1983) and should be investigated. Radical feminism posits that it is women, not men, who can be the knowers. Because women have been oppressed, they know more than men. They must see the world from the male perspective in order to survive, but their double vision from their experience as an oppressed group allows them to see more than men. In this respect radical feminism parallels Marxist feminist and African-American feminist critiques of who has the most accurate view of reality.

However, radical feminism deviates considerably from other feminisms in its view of how beliefs are legitimated as knowledge. A successful strategy that women use to obtain reliable knowledge and correct the distortions of patriarchal ideology is the consciousness-raising group (Jaggar, 1983). Using their personal experiences as a basis, women meet together in communal, nonhierarchical groups to examine their experiences to determine what counts as knowledge (MacKinnon, 1987).

The Boston Women's Health Book Collective and other women's health collectives serve as examples of women's attempts to understand their health experiences through a collective coming together. *Our Bodies, Ourselves* (1978, 1984, 1992) represents a product of their collective knowledge based on those experiences.

Because of the belief of radical feminists in connection and a conception of the world as an organic whole, they reject dualistic and hierarchical approaches. Dichotomies such as rational/feeling, objective/subjective, mind/body, culture/nature, and theory/practice are viewed as patriarchal conceptions which fragment the organic whole of reality. Holistic approaches without separations into mind/body and spiritual/physical parts become compatible with this connected approach to health. Linear conceptions of time and what is considered to be "logical" thinking in the Western traditions are frequently rejected by radical feminists. Cyclicity as a conception of time and thinking as an upward spiral seem more appropriate ways to study a world in which everything is connected in a process of constant change (Daly, 1978, 1984). Under radical feminism the female body, with its cyclicity of menstruation, serves as the ideal model for other nonreproductive hormones and continual biological change (Hoffman, 1982); the static male body is a deviation from the female norm.

Radical feminists view all human beings, and most particularly themselves, as connected to the living and nonliving world. Consequently, they view themselves as "participators" (Jaggar, 1983) connected in the same plane with, rather than distanced from, their object of study. Many radical feminists also believe that because of this connection, women can know things by relying on intuition and/or spiritual powers. Women's knowledge through experience of what is healthy would be viewed as superior to that of the male physician based on medical studies. Radical feminists vary in their belief as to whether the special ways of knowing of women are due to their biology (Daly, 1978; Griffin, 1978) or to their common social experiences as an oppressed group (Belenky et al., 1986) or both.

LESBIAN SEPARATISM

By its very nature, radical feminism emphasizes connection among the diverse beliefs held by women about ways to obtain knowledge and rejects the examination of a constantly changing, complex whole by looking at one of its parts. However, lesbian separatism, usually viewed as a subgroup theory within radical feminism, has some interesting implications for feminist methodology in science and medical research. To the tenets of radical feminist theory and their methodological implications for a feminist science, lesbian separatism provides one major addition. Lesbian separatists suggest that daily interaction with the patriarchal world and compulsory heterosexuality (Rich, 1976) make it impossible for women to understand completely their oppression and its distortion of their experience of reality. Therefore, in order to connect with other women and nature to understand reality, women must separate themselves from men. Only when freed from male oppression and patriarchy for a considerable period of time will women be able to understand their experiences and ways of knowing. Although based on separation from one part of reality—men—presumably lesbian separatists seek separation in order to enhance connection with the rest of reality. Radical feminism in general, and lesbian separatism in particular, suggest that their methods, arising from an extremely different view of reality, would result in a very different science, scientific method, and medicine.

Without obstetrics/gynecology and its emphasis upon procreation and heterosexual activity, research, diagnosis, and treatment in women's health might look quite different. The theory of separatism suggests the possible evolution of women-centered research agendas, created and carried out by female researchers using women as participant-subjects to develop health promotion and disease prevention for women in the absence of patriarchal hierarchies and strictures.

Given the current oppression of women and the male-dominated scientific and medical hierarchy which dictates the scientific problems considered worthy of funding for study and the acceptable approaches that might be used to study those problems, the results of a radical feminist science and health research agenda and especially of lesbian separatism are unimaginable.

There is certainly not just one feminist methodology, just as there is not one feminist theory. The jumble of descriptors for feminist method-ology—rejects dualisms, is based on women's experience, shortens the distance between observer and object of study, rejects unicausal, hierar-chical approaches, unites application with problem—may seem contra-dictory, but they become much more understandable when viewed as a lumping together of possible methodological implications for science and clinical research resulting from different feminist theories. This lumping together explains why some feminist theories (liberal and psychoanalytic) posit that feminist methodologies would lead to gender-free or gender-neutral research that could be carried out by male or female researchers, while others (essentialist and radical) suggest that only women could develop feminist methodologies for clinical research. Most feminist the-ories, with the exception of liberal feminism, reject the neutral objective observer for a social construction of scientific research based on the standpoint of the observer, which is influenced by gender, as well as other factors such as race and class. Radical feminism, and particularly lesbian separatism, suggest strong reasons for why we are not able to see the results of feminist methodologies. Implications of feminist methodologies serve as useful parameters for evaluating proposed changes in health care.

REFERENCES

Arnup, Katherine; Levesque, Andre; and Pierson, Ruth. 1990. *Delivering mother-hood: Maternal ideologies and practices in the nineteenth and twentieth centuries.* New York: Routledge.

Belenky, Mary Field; Clinchy, Blythe McVicker; Goldberger, Nancy Rule; and Tarule, Jill Mattuck. 1986. *Women's ways of knowing.* New York: Basic Books.

Biology and Gender Study Group. 1989. The importance of feminist critique for contemporary cell biology. In Nancy Tuana (ed.), *Feminism and science.* Bloomington: Indiana University Press.

Birke, Lynda. 1986. *Women, feminism, and biology: The feminist challenge.* New York: Methuen.

Blackwell, Antoinette. [1875] 1976. *The sexes throughout nature.* New York: G. P. Putnam's Sons. Reprint. Westport, Conn.: Hyperion Press, Inc.

Bleier, Ruth. 1979. Social and political bias in science: An examination of animal studies and their generalizations to human behavior and evolution. In Ruth Hubbard and Marian Lowe (eds.), *Genes and gender II: Pitfalls in research on sex and gender,* pp. 49–70. New York: Gordian Press.

———. 1984. *Science and gender: A critique of biology and its theories on women.* Elmsford, N.Y.: Pergamon Press.

———. 1986. Sex differences research: Science or belief? In Ruth Bleier (ed.), *Feminist approaches to science,* pp. 147–164. Elmsford, N.Y.: Pergamon Press.

————. 1988. Science and the construction of meanings in the neurosciences. In Sue V. Rosser (ed.), *Feminism within the science and health care professions: Overcoming resistance.* Elmsford, N.Y.: Pergamon Press.

Boston Women's Health Book Collective. 1978. *Our bodies, ourselves.* New York: Simon and Schuster. Revised and expanded 1984, 1992.

Buffery, W., and Gray, J. 1972. Sex differences in the development of spatial and linguistic skills. In C. Ounsted and D. C. Taylor (eds.), *Gender differences: Their ontogeny and significance.* Edinburg: Churchill Livingstone.

Calkins, M. W. 1896. Community of ideas of men and women. *Psychological Review* 3, no. 4:426–430.

Capra, Fritz. 1973. *The Tao of physics.* New York: Bantam Books.

Chasnoff, Ira J.; Landress, Harvey J.; and Barrett, Mark E. 1990. The prevalence of illicit-drug or alcohol abuse during pregnancy and discrepancies in mandated reporting in Pinellas County, Florida. *New England Journal of Medicine* 26 (April):1202.

Chodorow, Nancy. 1978. *The reproduction of mothering: Psychoanalysis and the sociology of gender.* Berkeley and Los Angeles: The University of California Press.

Corea, Gena. 1985. *The mother machine: Reproductive technologies from artificial insemination to artificial wombs.* New York: Harper and Row.

Daly, Mary. 1978. *Gyn/Ecology: The metaethics of radical feminism.* Boston: Beacon Press.

————. 1984. *Pure lust: Elemental feminist philosophy.* Boston: Beacon Press.

Dawkins, Richard. 1976. *The selfish gene.* New York: Oxford University Press.

de Beauvoir, Simone. 1974. *The second sex.* Trans. and ed. H. M. Parshley. New York: Vintage Books.

Dinnerstein, Dorothy. 1977. *The mermaid and the minotaur: Sexual arrangements and human malaise.* New York: Harper Colophon Books.

DuBois, Ellen, et al. 1985. *Feminist scholarship: Kindling in the groves of academe.* Urbana: University of Illinois Press.

Dworkin, Andrea. 1983. *Right-wing women.* New York: Coward-McCann.

Ehrenreich, Barbara, and English, Deirdre. 1978. *For her own good.* New York: Anchor Press.

Fausto-Sterling, Anne. 1985. *Myths of gender.* New York: Basic Books.

Fee, Elizabeth. 1982. A feminist critique of scientific objectivity. *Science for the People* 14, no. 4:8.

————. 1983. Women's nature and scientific objectivity. In Marian Lowe and Ruth Hubbard (eds.), *Women's nature: Rationalizations of inequality.* Elmsford, N.Y.: Pergamon Press.

Fennema, Elizabeth, and Sherman, Julie. 1977. Sex related differences in mathematics achievement, spatial visualization and affective factors. *American Educational Research Journal* 14:51–71.

Firestone, Shulamith. 1970. *The dialectic of sex.* New York: Bantam Books.

Flax, Jane. 1981. Do feminists need Marxism? *Building feminist theory: Essays from "Quest," A Feminist Quarterly,* pp. 174–185. New York: Longman.

Foreman, Ann. 1977. *Femininity as alienation: Women and the family in Marxism and psychoanalysis.* London: Pluto Press.

Fox-Genovese, Elizabeth. 1991. *Feminism without illusions.* Chapel Hill: University of North Carolina Press.

Friedan, Betty. 1974. *The feminine mystique.* New York: Dell.

Goldman, Emma. 1931. *Living my life.* 2 vols. New York: Alfred A. Knopf. Reprint. New York: Dover Publications, 1970.

Goodfield, June. 1981. *An imagined world.* New York: Penguin Books.

Gorski, Robert; Harlan, R. E.; Jacobson, C. D.; Shryne, J. E.; and Southam, A. M.

1980. Evidence for the existence of a sexually dimorphic nucleus in the preoptic area of the rat. *Journal of Comparative Neurology* 193:529–539.

Gould, Stephen Jay. 1981. *The mismeasure of man.* New York: W. W. Norton.

Goy, Robert, and Phoenix, C. H. 1971. The effects of testosterone propionate administered before birth on the development of behavior in genetic female rhesus monkeys. In C. H. Sawyer and R. A. Gorski (eds.), *Steroid hormones and brain function.* Berkeley: University of California Press.

Griffin, Susan. 1978. *Women and nature: The roaring inside her.* New York: Harper and Row.

Gurwitz, Jerry; Nananda, F. Colonel; and Avorn, Jerry. 1992. The exclusion of the elderly and women from clinical trials in acute myocardial infarction. *Journal of the American Medical Association* 268, no. 2:1407–1422.

Haraway, Donna. 1978. Animal sociology and a natural economy of the body politic, Part I: A political physiology of dominance; Animal sociology and a natural economy of the body politic, Part II: The past is the contested zone: Human nature and theories of production and reproduction in primate behavior studies. *Signs: Journal of Women in Culture and Society* 4, no. 1:21–60.

———. 1990. *Primate visions.* New York: Routledge.

Harding, Sandra. 1986. *The science question in feminism.* Ithaca, N.Y.: Cornell University Press.

———. 1987. *Feminism and methodology.* Bloomington and Indianapolis: Indiana University Press.

Hartman, Mary, and Banner, Lois (eds.). 1974. *Clio's consciousness raised.* New York.

Hartmann, Heidi. 1981. The unhappy marriage of Marxism and feminism: Towards a more progressive union. In Lydia Sargent (ed.), *Women and revolution: A discussion of the unhappy marriage of Marxism and feminism,* pp. 1–41. Boston: South End Press.

Hein, Hilde. 1981. Women and science: Fitting men to think about nature. *International Journal of Women's Studies* 4:369–377.

Hoffman, Joan. 1982. Biorhythms in human reproduction: The not-so-steady states. *Signs* 7, no. 4:829–844.

Hollingsworth, Leta S. 1914. Variability as related to sex differences in achievement. *American Journal of Sociology* 19, no. 4:510–530.

Hubbard, Ruth. 1979. Have only men evolved? In R. Hubbard, M. S. Henifin, and B. Fried (eds.), *Women look at biology looking at women.* Cambridge, Mass.: Schenkman.

———. 1990. *The politics of woman's biology.* New Brunswick, N.J.: Rutgers University Press.

Hubbard, Ruth, and Lowe, Marian. 1979. Introduction. In Ruth Hubbard and Marian Lowe (eds.), *Genes and gender II: Pitfalls in research on sex and gender.* New York: Gordian Press.

Hynes, H. Patricia. 1989. *The recurring silent spring.* Elmsford, N.Y.: Pergamon Press.

Jaggar, Alison M. 1983. *Feminist politics and human nature.* Totowa, N.J.: Rowman and Allanheld.

Jaggar, Alison, and Rothenberg, Paula (eds.). 1984. *Feminist frameworks.* New York: McGraw-Hill.

Johnson, Tracy L. 1993. A women's health research agenda. *Journal of Women's Health* 2, no. 2:95–98.

Jones, James. 1981. *Bad blood.* New York: Free Press.

Keller, Evelyn Fox. 1982. Feminism and Science. *Signs* 7, no. 3: 589–602.

———. 1983. *A feeling for the organism: The life and work of Barbara McClintock.* New York: W. H. Freeman.

————. 1984. Women and basic research: Respecting the unexpected. *Technology Review* (November/December):44–47.

————. 1985. *Reflections on gender and science.* New Haven, Conn.: Yale University Press.

————. 1987. Women scientists and feminist critics of science. *Daedalus* 116, no. 4:77–91.

Kelsey, Sheryl, et al. 1993. *Circulation* (March).

Kuhn, Thomas S. 1970. *The structure of scientific revolutions.* 2nd ed. Chicago: University of Chicago Press.

Lancaster, Jane. 1975. *Primate behavior and the emergence of human culture.* New York: Holt, Rinehart and Winston.

Leavitt, Ruth R. 1975. *Peaceable primates and gentle people: Anthropological approaches to women's studies.* New York: Harper and Row.

Leibowitz, Lila. 1975. Perspectives in the evolution of sex differences. In R. R. Reiter (ed.), *Toward an anthropology of women.* New York: Monthly Review Press.

MacKinnon, Catharine. 1982. Feminism, Marxism, method and the state: An agenda for theory. *Signs: Journal of Women in Culture and Society* 7, no. 3:515–544.

MacKinnon, Catharine A. 1987. *Feminism unmodified: Discourses on life and law.* Cambridge, Mass., and London: Harvard University Press.

Merchant, Carolyn. 1979. *The death of nature: Women, ecology and the scientific revolution.* New York: Harper and Row.

Mill, Harriet Taylor. 1970. Enfranchisement of women. In Alice S. Rossi (ed.), *Essays on sex equality.* Chicago: University of Chicago Press.

Mill, John Stuart. 1970 The subjection of women. In John Stuart Mill and Harriet Taylor Mill, *Essays on sex equality,* ed. Alice S. Rossi, pp. 123–242. Chicago: University of Chicago Press.

Millett, Kate. 1970. *Sexual politics.* Garden City, N.Y.: Doubleday.

Mitchell, Juliet. 1971. *Woman's estate.* New York: Pantheon Books.

————. 1974. *Psychoanalysis and feminism.* New York: Vintage Books.

National Science Foundation. 1990. *Women and minorities in science and engineering.* NSF 90–301. Washington, D.C.: Author.

O'Brien, Mary. 1981. *The politics of reproduction.* Boston: Routledge and Kegan Paul.

Ortner, Sherry. 1974. Is female to male as nature to culture? In Michelle Rosaldo and Louise Lamphere (eds.), *Woman, culture, and society.* Stanford: Stanford University Press.

Rich, Adrienne. 1976. *Of woman born: Motherhood as experience.* New York: W. W. Norton.

Rosser, Sue V. 1982. Androgyny and sociobiology. *International Journal of Women's Studies* 5, no. 5:435–444.

————. 1988. Women in science and health care: A gender at risk. In Sue V. Rosser (ed.), *Feminism within the science and health care professions: Overcoming resistance.* Elmsford, N.Y.: Pergamon Press.

————. 1990. *Female-friendly science.* Elmsford, N.Y.: Pergamon Press.

Rossiter, Margaret W. 1982. *Women scientists in America: Struggles and strategies to 1940.* Baltimore, Md.: The Johns Hopkins University Press.

Rowell, Thelma. 1974. The concept of social dominance. *Behavioral Biology* 11:131–154.

Sayers, Janet. 1982. *Biological politics: Feminist and anti-feminist perspectives.* London: Tavistock.

Section for Student Services. 1992. In Janet Bickel and Renee Quinnie (eds.),

Women in medicine statistics. Washington, D.C.: Association of American Medical Colleges.

Sherman, Elizabeth; Johnson, David; and Whiting, Brooke. 1990. *Participation of women and minorities on US Medical school faculties 1980–1990.* Washington, D.C.: Association of American Medical Colleges.

Smith-Rosenberg, Carol. 1975. The female world of love and ritual: Relations between women in nineteenth century America. *Signs* 1 (Autumn):1–29.

Spanier, Bonnie. 1982. Toward a balanced curriculum: The study of women at Wheaton College. *Change* 14 (April):31–34.

Sperry, R. W. 1974. Lateral specialization in the surgically separated hemispheres. In F. O. Schmitt and R. T. Wardon, *The neurosciences: Third study program.* Cambridge: MIT Press.

Star, Susan Leigh. 1979. Sex differences and the dichotomization of the brain: Methods, limits and problems in research on consciousness. In Ruth Hubbard and Marian Lowe (eds.), *Genes and gender II: Pitfalls in research on sex and gender.* New York: Gordian Press.

Steering Committee on the Physician's Health Study Group. 1989. Final report of the aspirin component of the ongoing Physician's Health Study. *New England Journal of Medicine* 3221:129–135.

Sullivan, Deborah, and Weitz, Rose. 1988. *Labor pains: Modern midwives and home birth.* New Haven, Conn.: Yale University Press.

Tanner, A. 1896. The community of ideas of men and women. *Psychological Review* 3, no. 5:548–550.

Tong, Rosemarie. 1989. *Feminist thought: A comprehensive introduction.* Boulder: Westview Press.

Trivers, Robert L. 1972. Parental investment and sexual selection. In B. Campbell (ed.), *Sexual selection and the descent of man.* Chicago: Aldine.

U.S. General Accounting Office. National Institutes of Health: Problems in implementing policy on women in study populations. Statement of Mark V. Nadel, Associate Director, National and Public Health Issues, Human Resources Division, before the Subcommittee on Health and the Environment, Committee on Energy and Commerce, U.S. House of Representatives, June 19, 1990.

Vetter, Betty. 1988. Where are the women in the physical sciences? In Sue V. Rosser (ed.), *Feminism within the science and health care professions: Overcoming resistance.* New York: Pergamon Press.

Vogel, Lise. 1983. *Marxism and the oppression of women: Towards a unitary theory.* New Brunswick, N.J.: Rutgers University Press.

Wertz, Richard, and Wertz, Dorothy. 1977. *Lying-in: A history of childbirth in America.* New York: Schocken Books.

Wilson, Edward O. 1975. *Sociobiology: The new synthesis.* Cambridge, Mass.: Harvard University Press.

Wollstonecraft, Mary. 1975. *A vindication of the rights of woman.* Ed. Carol H. Poston. New York: W. W. Norton.

Yerkes, R. M. 1943. *Chimpanzees.* New Haven: Yale University Press.

Young, Iris. 1980. Socialist feminism and the limits of dual systems theory. *Socialist Review* 10, nos. 2–3:174.

———. 1981. Beyond the unhappy marriage: A critique of the dual systems theory. In Lydia Sargent (ed.), *Women and revolution: A discussion of the unhappy marriage of Marxism and feminism.* Boston: South End Press.

CHAPTER NINE

More Than "Add Women and Stir"

Integrating Disease and Health of Women into the Medical Curriculum

Following closely on the heels of the widespread acknowledgment that women and their health have been excluded, overlooked, and understudied has come the inevitable debate concerning how women should be included in the medical profession and curriculum. A recent focus of the debate is whether a separate specialty in women's health should be created, as opposed to incorporating women's health into existing specialties and curricula. The *Journal of Women's Health* featured a point/counterpoint discussion of this debate in its Summer 1992 issue.

Karen Johnson (1992) presented the case for a separate specialty in her article "Pro: Women's Health: Developing a New Interdisciplinary Specialty." Johnson succinctly summarizes her argument:

What most opponents fail to appreciate is that women's health is a unique body of knowledge and skills based upon experience with women that cross the boundaries of existing specialties. Women's health care needs are not being met, and cannot be met, within the existing medical paradigm. . . . I am hard pressed to understand why a specialty embracing 52% of the adult population is unreasonable or unnecessary. . . . Women deserve no less than children who have specialists in pediatrics and the elderly who have specialists in geriatrics. (P. 98)

Michelle Harrison (1992) argued against a new specialty in "Con: Women's Health as a Specialty: A Deceptive Solution." She opposes the idea, fearing it would lead to a new ghetto in women's health in addition to obstetrics/gynecology, which would again relieve general medicine and other specialties from including women in their central focus. Harrison eloquently states her objections to the specialty on those grounds:

The designation of obstetrics and gynecology as *the* women's specialty may have actually isolated the understanding of interrelations between menstruation, pregnancy, and other metabolic processes. And, because of bifurcation in treatment and approach to women's health, the rest of medicine has tended to leave these questions to obstetrics and gynecology. (P. 104)

Just recently in this century women have entered into medicine in significant numbers. However, their continued inability to achieve positions of power makes it likely that "women's health" would become a marginalized area for a few dedicated (probably mostly female) physicians. Meanwhile, the rest of medicine would continue as it is, with both the male body and the male psyche the standard of normality and health. And, as long as the standard is male, "other" invariably will mean less. (P. 105)

Her arguments have merit and seem reasonable, particularly in light of the history of medicine, the majority status of women in the population, and the difficulties surrounding the notion of "separate but equal." Lila Wallis suggested the merits and possible pitfalls of each stance in "Commentary: Women's Health: A Specialty? Pros and Cons." She concluded, "Both authors are right. The path of American medicine should take us to their recommendations one at a time" (Wallis, 1992, p. 108).

This debate is not unique to the area of women's health. It arises each time a body of new research approaches and theories of significance comes to the forefront and challenges the existing disciplines and structures of academia to accommodate it. Since the current organization of knowledge and disciplines evolved without this new field, it is not surprising that each new area does not easily fit into the existing structure of knowledge and disciplines.

The history of academia abounds with struggles to establish new fields and disciplines. During the eighteenth century, the social sciences fought to become respected areas of intellectual pursuit within universities basing their divisions on the traditional models of letters and sciences (Gordon, 1991; Ross, 1991). Within the social sciences, individual disciplines such as sociology (R. M. Williams, 1976) battled the more entrenched social science disciplines of economics, political science, and psychology for recognition as a distinct area of expertise. The history of medicine (Ehrenreich and English, 1979) reveals a similar struggle for emergence of specialties. Each of the specialties fought to distinguish itself as a separate entity from general medicine and from the existing specialties. The interdisciplinary specialties, subspecialties, and additional qualifications such as pediatrics and gerontology, distinguished by the age of the patient rather than basis in an organ or system, struggled with particular difficulty for establishment and recognition.

THE EXAMPLE OF WOMEN'S STUDIES

As each new field or specialty emerged, scholars and practitioners from traditional fields questioned its necessity. Couldn't these new ideas, approaches, or population needs simply be accommodated by a broadening of or reeducation of scholars and practitioners within currently existing disciplines or fields? Considerable division occurred a decade ago among investigators evolving the new scholarship on women about whether separate interdisciplinary programs or departments in women's studies should be created or whether scholars should incorporate women into the traditional disciplines (Arch and Kirschner, 1984; Bowles and Klein, 1983; Bunch and Pollack, 1983).

More than ten years after the initial autonomy-versus-integration debates in women's studies, almost no discussion centers on this issue. It no longer remains a controversial topic because the solution in most institutions was both to establish autonomous women's studies programs and to integrate the new scholarship on women into traditional disciplines. Using foundation and federal money, a few institutions (McMillen, 1987) tried integration in the absence of an established women's studies program. They discovered quickly that it was virtually impossible to sustain because they lacked the resources of faculty in women's studies knowledgeable about how to deal with difficulties, expand to new sources, and move on to the next phase after a relatively superficial introduction to curriculum integration.

For somewhat different reasons, institutions which developed departments of women's studies that for structural or ideological reasons made few attempts at integrating scholarship on women into the rest of the curriculum were usually less successful than those attempting to integrate in the presence of a strong program. Programs in women's studies adhering too closely to the autonomous model tended to have difficulties obtaining approval for women's studies majors, minors, graduate programs, and cross-listing courses, as well as having an impact on the broader curriculum. Because they had not reached out and attempted to integrate, their colleagues did not understand women's studies and were suspicious of it. Those institutions which most successfully integrated the new scholarship on women into the traditional disciplines did so in the presence of a strong women's studies program.

The debate over a specialty in women's health might profit from the example of women's studies in dealing with these similar issues. In addition to having evolved relatively recently, women's studies also centers on information about women. The same questions about the history of women in higher education, the majority status of women in the population, and "separate but equal" were considered and resolved in the autonomy-versus-integration debate within women's studies.

A MODEL FOR TRANSFORMATION

Institutions successful in transforming the curriculum to include women's studies developed the phase models and interactive roles for their new programs in the process. More than two decades of women's studies scholarship and experience with curriculum transformation projects have enabled faculty to develop models (McIntosh, 1984; Schuster and Van Dyne, 1985; Tetreault, 1985; Rosser, 1990) tracing the stages in a variety of disciplines in diverse institutions. All the models reflect the idea that integrating information about women into the curriculum is a process that occurs in phases. In the first phase, women are absent from the curriculum; the final phase is the gender-balanced curriculum. The model developed by Peggy McIntosh (1984) of the Wellesley Center for Research on Women will be elaborated and expanded here to illustrate the process of transforming the curriculum, using examples from five disciplines.

Phase I: The Womanless Curriculum

This is the traditional curricular approach in which the absence of women is not noted. In history it provides an exclusive approach to the discipline, in that only great events and men in history (i.e., presidents and battles) are deemed worthy of consideration. Art history courses recently taught on many campuses emphasize this phase. The most widely used art history text, by Janson, a very thick volume, included no women and no African-American artists until the 1986 edition (McNamee and Fix, 1986). English courses at this stage include no or very few women authors. Much psychological research and many psychology courses also exemplify this stage. For example, many theories of human development are really based on white male development. Levinson's model of adult development (1974), Erikson's model (1963), and of course Freud's work all assumed a male norm. In most biology and other science courses, gender is not even considered to be an issue, since science is objective.

Phase II: Women as an Add-on to the Curriculum

Heroines, exceptional women, or an elite few who are seen to have been of benefit to culture as defined by the traditional (white, male, middle/upper-class) standards of the discipline are included in the course of study at this stage. History courses might cover women such as Joan of Arc, Abigail Adams, or Betsy Ross. An art history course in phase II might include a few slides of work by Berthe Morisot or Mary Cassatt or a handout about them used with the Janson text. The first edition of the traditional Norton anthology in English included only two women, Jane Austen and Emily Dickinson; now in its fifth edition, as a result of the new scholarship on women, the anthology has evolved to include twenty-eight female authors. In psychology, the work of Melanie Klein, Karen Horney, or even Anna Freud, who modified Freud's ideas about women, might be characterized as being at this stage. Science courses that emphasize the nine women who have won the Nobel Prize in medicine or science would certainly be categorized here. In phase II, women are added on without a change in the basic syllabus or traditional framework of the course.

Phase III: Women as a Problem, Anomaly, or Absence from the Curriculum

Women are studied in this phase as victims, as deprived or defective variants of men, or as protesters, with issues. Scholars begin to view gender as intersecting with race and class to form complex interlocking political phenomena.

At this phase, historians may begin to ask why there have been no women presidents. People considering art history begin to ask questions such as, Why aren't there more women and people of color labeled as artists—and what is art, anyway? In English the question becomes, Why aren't there any female Shakespeares? In psychology the issue is why women's development doesn't fit the model of human development. This soon leads to the question of what must be wrong with models that don't fit the development of more than half of the people in the world since they don't fit women and men of color or white women. Many biologists at this stage point out flaws in experimental design in some of the studies which have supposedly "proven" superior mathematical ability in males. They also question the circularity of logic involved in some sociobiology research in which human language and frameworks are used to describe certain animal behaviors such as aggression, which is then used to prove that certain human behavior is biologically determined, since it has also been found in animals.

Phase IV: Women as the Focus for Studies

In this phase the categories for analysis shift and become racially inclusive, multifaceted, and filled with variety; they demonstrate and validate plural versions of reality.

This phase takes account of the fact that since women have had half of the world's lived experience, we need to ask what that experience has been and to consider it as half of history. This causes faculty to utilize all kinds of evidence and source materials which academic people are not in the habit of using. People doing art history research at this phase may begin to look at certain types of crafts, quilts, and stitchery work (much of which has traditionally been done by women and people of color) as art. In English people look at women's writing—diaries, letters, novels. They examine it both for what it is and for how it differs from that of men. Psychologists such as Carol Gilligan (1982) have begun to explore female models of development which emphasize different methods of ethical and moral decision-making practiced by girls and women.

In biology the work of Barbara McClintock may serve as an example of this stage of research. In her approach toward studying maize, she indicated a shortening of the distance between the observer and the object being studied and a consideration of the complex interaction between the organism and its environment.

Phase V: The Curriculum Redefined and Reconstructed to Include Us All

The ultimate goal is a gender-balanced curriculum. Although this course of study will be a long time in the making, it will help students to see that women are both part of and alien to the dominant culture. It will create more usable and inclusive constructs which validate a broader spectrum of life with regard to race, class, and gender.

Phase V is the goal toward which women's studies strives. In this final phase women are not separated out but are present in all disciplines; the womanless curriculum has not been replaced by the manless curriculum. Knowledge about women, race, and class is present in all introductory and advanced courses.

APPLICATION OF THE MODEL TO A SPECIALTY IN WOMEN'S HEALTH

Aside from the wars and battles over money triggered by the proposal for any new specialty (Task Force, 1992), particularly in these tight fiscal times, few would question the need for a specialty which by definition would serve 52 percent of the adult population. It is precisely the fact that women would serve as the focus that makes many individuals, including many female physicians, question the advisability of a separate specialty. They note that male physicians seized control of childbirth from female midwives and defined it as a surgical specialty (Ehrenreich and English, 1979). The creation of the specialty of obstetrics/gynecology led to a loss of attention to women's health concerns other than reproduction. They are aware that this bifurcation in the system, while officially relegating only some aspects of women's health to obstetrics/gynecology, in reality meant that general medicine and the other specialties focused only on the male. Women and their health problems were thereby virtually excluded from research agendas in all areas of medicine except obstetrics/gynecology.

Despite these complications, women's studies phase theory suggests a model in which both a specialty in women's health and inclusion of women's health in general medicine and other medical specialties might evolve to mutually reinforce each other. Although presented as distinct stages, the phases in this model should be visualized as a continuous upward spiral.

Phase I: Absence of Women and Women's Health Is Not Noted

By and large, this phase describes the status of most medical research and medical curricula before the late 1980s.

Research: Before an audit by the General Accounting Office drew attention to the exclusion of women as experimental subjects from research protocols in studies funded by NIH, the omission of women from research protocols was rarely noted (*National News and Development*, 1986). Congress, led by women such as Pat Schroeder and Barbara Mikulski, began to question the absence of substantial research devoted to women's health concerns at that time and to lead the fight for funding and focus on such research on the national level.

Curriculum: The lecturer who uses without question the 70 kilogram male as the norm and emphasis on diagnosis and disease processes as they occur in the white man's body (without stating explicitly that this is the perspective from which the course is taught) exemplifies this phase in the medical curriculum. The specialty of obstetrics/gynecology and the illusion that this specialty includes women's health beyond the reproductive system made the absence of women and women's health from the rest of the medical curriculum pass without notice or seem reasonable when questioned.

Phase II: Add-and-Stir Approaches to Women and Women's Health Are Attempted

Even before the attention drawn by Congress and the NIH to the absence of women, many researchers, teachers, and practitioners became aware that their experimental designs, explanations, and diagnoses suffered from the exclusion of women. They sought to remedy the situation by adding women on to the existing experimental protocol or explication. At this phase, the question was not raised whether the experimental design, lecture, or procedure might need to be modified because of the addition of women; women were simply added to experiments and explanations developed using the male as norm.

Research: Phase II research is exemplified by some of the 18 percent of clinical trials between 1960 and 1991 for medications to prevent myocardial infarctions (Gurwitz, Nananda, and Avorn, 1992) which included women but used subjects less than seventy-five years old. By using women and men of the same age, these studies assumed the male norm for myocardial infarction. They failed to take into account its later onset in women, who constitute 24 percent of those younger than sixty-five and 64 percent of those at age eighty-five or older who die of acute myocardial infarction (Kapantis and Powell-Griner, 1989). By choosing the male body as the norm for the experiment and simply adding women subjects, these experiments fed the myth of heart disease as a male disease, rather than revealing the fact that heart disease strikes men and women with similar frequencies but at different ages.

Curriculum: Faculty often present lectures at the phase II stage. After explaining anatomy, physiology, or disease processes using the male body as the norm, the faculty member may note a slight variation that occurs in females, without explaining its possible implications or ramifications. For example, in a lecture on the use of oral antibiotics such as penicillin to fight streptococcus infections in the throat, the lecturer might note that women may experience vaginal yeast infections after using the antibiotics. If the lecturer fails to explain that the oral administration of the antibiotic kills bacteria all over the body, not just in the throat, the source of the yeast infection may not be understood. The lecturer also misses an opportunity to explain the mechanism by which bacteria and yeast normally function to limit each other's growth in the vaginal area.

Phase III: Women Are Seen as a Problem, Anomaly, or Deviant from the Norm

By this phase, investigators and teachers recognize that simply adding women and women's health to research and lectures designed using the white male as the standard of normality often yields only inadequate, partial explanations for women.

Research: Cardiac researchers at this phase couple this recognition with the obvious statistical evidence that women live an average of 7.5 years longer than men (National Center for Health Statistics, 1992), and that heart disease is the major killer of older women. This enables these investigators to rethink experimental protocols. They begin to question including only males under the age of seventy-five as subjects for myocardial infarction experiments and begin to explore the flaws introduced into experiments when variables such as gender, age, and menstrual status are not included in experimental design.

Curriculum: Instructing students in gross anatomy to cut off the breasts of female cadavers and discard them constitutes a most dramatic example of phase III teaching in the classroom (Lewin, 1992). As Dr. Fugh Berman asked: "How many . . . students . . . take away the message that despite the epidemic of breast cancer, women's breasts had no medical significance?" (Lewin, 1992, p. A-1). Lectures on AIDS diagnosis using the revised Centers for Disease Control (CDC, 1987) surveillance case definition predating the January 1993 revised definition also exemplify phase III classroom teaching. From their own practice, reading, and anecdotal information learned from colleagues, most faculty knew that the earlier revised CDC definition (CDC, 1987) was inadequate for diagnosing AIDS in women. The most evident problem was the omission of gynecologic conditions and their numerous complications—higher rates of cervical cancer, abnormal Pap smears, increased incidence of pelvic inflammatory disease, and vaginal infections resistant to cure—thought to be manifestations of the disease in women. Since the revised definition included no gynecologic conditions, women were seen as a problem or anomaly for AIDS diagnosis.

Phase IV: Women as the Focus

Once the pervasiveness of women's exclusion from research designs and curricula and the bias that exclusion introduces into research, teaching, and practice are understood, women become a new focal point for research and curricula.

Research: By this phase, a substantial group of investigators, lecturers, and practitioners evolve who commit their efforts and careers to studying women. These individuals design experiments which not only include women as experimental subjects but for which women's health, diseases, and issues also serve as the central topic of study. The topics lead to the development of experimental methods particularly appropriate for the female body and life cycle and the experiences of women. Race and class are understood to be interlocking phenomena with gender in the health and disease of women, which must also be integrated into research design, teaching, and practice.

Phase IV is the stage at which some forward-looking national leaders thinking about women's health currently find themselves. The establishment of the Office on Women's Health Research within NIH (1990) and the Women's Health Initiative (Healy, 1992) demonstrate early efforts to place women's health in central focus. The collection of baseline data sought in the Women's Health Initiative on the three major causes of death and frailty in women aged forty-five years and older—"cardiovascular diseases, cancers of the breast, lung, and colorectal tract, and osteoporosis" (Pinn and LaRosa, 1992)—underlines the extent to which the absence of women has not been noted previously in research and curricula in specialties outside of obstetrics/gynecology. Because obstetrics/gynecology is a surgical specialty which revolves around women of reproductive age and issues of reproduction, particularly sexually transmitted diseases, contraception, infertility, pregnancy, childbirth, and menopause, this information has not been collected and explored by researchers or practitioners in the field. Women are the primary focus of study under the Women's Health Initiative designed to collect these data and stimulate further research on cardiovascular disease, cancers, and osteoporosis.

Curriculum: A focus on women and their health is also beginning to be found at various levels of medical curricula. At Yale, the departments of medicine and obstetrics/gynecology have developed a program in women's health; the goals include a clinical model in women's health, a curriculum in women's health studies, and a center for research on women's health issues (Henrich, 1992). At the University of Louisville, faculty expose medical students to women's health issues at a Health Awareness Workshop Orientation prior to the onset of the first year of medical school, to a core lecture and elective on the new psychology of women and men in the sophomore year, and to a core lecture on psychiatry rotation and gender issues in medical practice in the junior year (Dickstein, 1992). The School of Medicine at SUNY–Stony Brook includes three foci for formal teaching specifically related to women in its "Medicine and Contemporary Society" class (120 hours during the first two years): women as patients, gender and the provision of health care, and women as physicians (P. C. Williams, 1992). In 1993, Stanford will undertake a program to develop curriculum-change proposals to train junior and senior medical faculty on the sociocultural, economic, and political factors that affect research and practice in women's health (Matteo, 1992).

In August 1992, the American Medical Women's Association (AMWA) held a retreat attended by twenty-eight women's health experts and official representatives of fifteen medical specialty societies. At the retreat, AMWA presented its Advanced Women's Health Curriculum targeted at physicians, particularly primary care physicians. Structured along the life cycle of women, the proposed curriculum includes a finite number of courses. Successful completion of the entire program coupled with the passing of a rigorous examination would lead to CME units and a certificate of completion of the Advanced Curriculum in Women's Health (Wallis, 1992).

These courses, residencies, and continuing medical education curricula represent initial attempts to focus on women's health at all levels of the medical curriculum. Coupled with the new research initiatives, they substantiate the need for a specialty in women's health. The individuals who develop and enhance the new research and curricula must be properly trained in order to advance this interdisciplinary field to phase V.

Phase V: Research and Curricula to Include Us All

The ultimate goal of a specialty in women's health is to integrate the information on women's health into research in all specialties and to transform all aspects of the medical curriculum to include women and their health. Patterned on women's studies and the Office of Research on Women's Health at NIH, the specialty would aid other disciplines and specialties in understanding the importance of including women in research and teaching while simultaneously providing trained specialists to undertake more focused research in this interdisciplinary field. A separate specialty or additional qualification in women's health would encourage general medicine and each of the other specialties to go through each of the above transformation phases until women and women's health are fully integrated into their research, teaching, and practice. Far from creating a ghetto, this phase model of the both/and approach demonstrates that a specialty in women's health would ensure the inclusion of women in all aspects of medicine.

One reason that proponents of each new field fight particularly hard for a new discipline or specialty is their recognition that traditional disciplines accommodate and integrate new information, theories, and approaches most effectively when forced by a distinct presence. In other words, in the absence of a separate specialty, traditional fields are less likely to perceive the information as important material to accommodate. A specialty provides the resources in terms of both research and practice for the information to be integrated into other aspects of medicine. Practitioners of the specialty recognize when their discoveries might be examined and used by other specialties and bring those discoveries to the attention of their colleagues in other disciplines. In the absence of a separate specialty and its associated researchers and practitioners, information from the new area is less likely to come to the attention of and be accommodated by the current researchers and practitioners of the traditional divisions of knowledge.

The answer to the debate over whether a women's health specialty or integration of more information about women's health into currently existing specialties and general medicine is needed is yes, both/and. An interdisciplinary specialty in women's health must be created to serve as a source of research and information that can be used to transform other areas of medicine to include and apply this information. In addition to defining the research for the specialty, research specialists and practitioners in women's health can guide their colleagues in other branches of medicine in this transformation. Handling problems that cross boundaries of current specialties, practitioners of women's health can refer patients to another appropriate specialty when the problem is not addressed better by the new interdisciplinary specialty.

REFERENCES

Arch, Elizabeth, and Kirschner, Susan. 1984. Transformation of the curriculum: Problems of conception and deception. *Women's Studies International Forum* 3:149.

Bowles, Gloria, and Klein, Renate D. 1983. *Theories of women's studies.* London: Routledge and Kegan Paul.

Bunch, Charlotte, and Pollack, Sandra. 1983. *Learning our way: Essays in feminist education.* Trumansburg, N.Y.: The Crossing Press.

Centers for Disease Control. 1987. Revision of the CDC surveillance case definition for acquired immunodeficiency syndrome. *Morbidity and Mortality Weekly Report* 35:15.

Dickstein, Leah. 1992. Women's health curricula at the University of Louisville School of Medicine. Reframing Women's Health: Multidisciplinary Research and Practice Conference, October 15–17 workshop abstracts. Chicago: University of Illinois at Chicago Center for Research on Women and Gender.

Ehrenreich, Barbara, and English, Deirdre. 1979. *For her own good: 150 years of the experts' advice to women.* Garden City, N.Y.: Anchor Books.

Erikson, Erik H. 1963. *Childhood and society.* 2nd ed. New York: Norton.

Gilligan, Carol. 1982. *In a different voice.* Cambridge, Mass.: Harvard University Press.

Gordon, S. 1991. Sociality and social science. In *The history and philosophy of social science.* New York: Routledge.

Gurwitz, Jerry H.; Nananda, F. Colonel; and Avorn, Jerry. The exclusion of the elderly and women from clinical trials in acute myocardial infarctions. *Journal of the American Medical Association* 11:1417.

Harrison, Michelle. 1992. Con: Women's health as a specialty: A deceptive solution. *Journal of Women's Health* 2:101.

Healy, Bernadine. 1992. Women's health, public welfare. *Journal of the American Medical Association* 4:566.

Henrich, Janet. 1992. The program in women's health at Yale. Presented at Reframing Women's Health: Multidisciplinary Research and Practice Conference, October 15–17 workshop abstracts. Chicago: University of Illinois at Chicago Center for Research on Women and Gender.

Johnson, Karen. 1992. Pro: Women's health: Developing a new interdisciplinary specialty. *Journal of Women's Health* 2:101.

Kapantis, G., and Powell-Griner, G. 1989. *Characteristics of persons dying of disease of the heart: Preliminary data from the 1986 National Mortality Followback Survey.* Hyattsville, Md.: National Center for Health Statistics.

Keller, Evelyn F. 1984. Women and the basic research: Respecting the unexpected. *Technology Review,* November/December 1984, pp. 44–47.

Levinson, D. J.; Darrow, C. M.; Klein, E. B.; Levinson, M. H.; and McKee, B. 1974. The psychosocial development of men in early adulthood and the mid-life transition. In D. F. Ricks, A. Thomas, and M. Roff (eds.), *Life history research in psychotherapy 3.* Minneapolis: University of Minnesota Press.

Lewin, T. 1992. Doctors consider a specialty focusing on women's health. *The New York Times,* November 7, p. A-1.

Matteo, S. 1992. Women, gender and the medical curriculum: Building a new educational paradigm. Reframing Women's Health: Multidisciplinary Research and Practice Conference, October 15–17 workshop abstracts. Chicago: University of Illinois at Chicago Center for Research on Women and Gender.

McIntosh, P. 1984. The study of women: Processes of personal and curricular re-vision. *The Forum for Liberal Education* 5:2.

McMillen, Wendy. 1987. More colleges and more disciplines incorporating scholarship on women into the classroom. *The Chronicle of Higher Education* 34:A15–17.

McNamee, Harriot, and Fix, Dorothy. 1986. Art workshop. In S. Coulter, K. Edgington, and E. Hedges (eds.), *Resources for curriculum change.* Towson, Md.: Towson State University.

National Center for Health Statistics. 1992. *Vital statistics of the United States* 2 (ptA). Washington, D.C.: Public Health Service.

National News and Development. 1986. NIH urges inclusion of women in clinical study populations. 52:2.

Pinn, Vivian, and LaRosa, Judith. 1992. *Overview: Office of research on women's health.* Bethesda, Md.: National Institutes of Health.

Ross, D. 1991. The discovery of modernity. In *The origins of American social science.* New York: Cambridge University Press.

Rosser, Sue V. 1990. *Female-friendly science.* Elmsford, N.Y.: Pergamon Press.

Schuster, Marilyn R., and Van Dyne, Susan. 1985. *Women's place in the academy: Transforming the liberal arts curriculum.* Totowa, N.J.: Rowman and Allanheld.

Skolnick, A. 1992. Women's health specialty, other issues on agenda of 'Reframing' conference. *Journal of the American Medical Association* 14:1813.

Task Force on the Generalist Physician. 1992. Executive summary. Washington, D.C.: Association of American Medical Colleges.

Tetreault, Mary K. 1985. Stages of thinking about women: An experience-derived evaluation model. *The Journal of Higher Education* 5:368–384.

Wallis, Lila. 1992. Commentary: Women's health: A specialty? Pros and cons. *Journal of Women's Health* 2:107.

Wallis, Lila A. 1992. Women's health curriculum abstract for Reframing Women's Health: Multidisciplinary Research and Practice Conference, October 15–17 workshop abstracts. Chicago: University of Illinois at Chicago Center for Research on Women and Gender.

Williams, P. C. 1992. Focus on women's health at SUNY–Stony Brook. *Women in Medicine Update* 6, no. 4:1–2.

Williams, R. M. 1976. Sociology in America. In C. Bonjean, L. Schneider, and R. L. Lineberry (eds.), *Social science in America.* Austin: University of Texas Press.

CHAPTER TEN

A Chilly Climate for Women in Medicine

During the past two decades, American medicine has witnessed a dramatic change in the gender composition of the classes graduating from medical school. In 1969–70, women constituted 8.4 percent of medical school graduates; by 1989–90 that figure had risen to 34.5 percent (Bickel and Quinnie, 1992). The upward trend continues for the foreseeable future, as women made up 41.6 percent of the new entrants in 1992–93 (Section for Student Services, 1992).

The pool of physicians also becomes more diverse with regard to factors other than gender with each passing decade. Although increases in racial diversity have not occurred as rapidly as the increase in the number of women, medical students are more racially diverse than they were two decades ago. In 1992 (Section for Student Services, 1992), 1,273 of 15,365 (8.3 percent) medical school graduates fell into the category of underrepresented minorities (Black, American Indian/Alaska Native, Mexican-American/Chicano, Puerto Rican, Mainland Puerto Rican). Underrepresented minorities constituted 1,827 of 16,289, or 11.2 percent, of all new entrants to medical school in 1992–93 (Section for Student Services, 1992); this figure contrasts with the 1968–69 figure of 3 percent (Jolly, 1993). A higher proportion of underrepresented minority 1992 graduates (660) and 1992–93 new entrants (1,017) were women, compared to men graduates (613) and new male entrants (810) that year (Section for Student Services, 1992).

Current medical school classes are also less homogeneous with regard to age. The average age of medical students has changed considerably during the last twenty years; the women are somewhat older than the men students (Bickel and Quinnie, 1992). Entrants to medical school now begin with more debt and graduate with more debts to repay than their predecessors. Male students begin medical school with slightly more educational debt ($9,057) than female students ($8,510) (Bickel, 1992). But women hold more consumer debt upon entrance ($17,060) than men students ($12,612). Women also come from parental families with lower incomes ($81,329) compared to men students ($86,933), and are married to spouses with higher debt ($13,517) than that of wives of male medical students ($9,687) (Bickel, 1992).

The increases in numbers of women, racial diversity, age, and indebtedness of current medical students reflect trends in the American population overall, which is older, more racially diverse, carries more debt, and has a much higher percentage of women in the workforce than two decades ago. Projections based upon the demographic composition of the United States and its relative position in the world economy suggest that these trends will continue to increase at a more rapid rate into the twenty-first century.

> The composition of the workforce in the year 2000 is projected to be quite different from what we have today. There will be a larger segment of minorities and women: 23 percent more Blacks, 70 percent more Asians and other races (American Indians, Alaska natives and Pacific Islanders), 74 percent more Hispanics and 25 percent more women adding 3.6 million, 2.4 million, 6.0 million and 13.0 million more workers respectively. Altogether, the minorities and women will make up 90 percent of the workforce growth and 23 percent of the new employees will be immigrants. (Thomas, 1989, p. 30)

Since women and minorities represent the sectors of workforce growth, future medical classes must also reflect increasing racial diversity and include larger numbers of women. Unfortunately, the structures of medical education, hospital and clinical practices, informal and formal policies, and medical leaders have changed much more slowly than the demographic composition of the medical school classes.

For decades white men have dominated the medical profession. While rigorous and grueling, medical school, residency, and the practice of medicine were not impossible or even incompatible with the lifestyle of a white male whose income as a physician could support a wife to stay at home and take care of the children and household duties. As women, men of color, older people, less affluent individuals, and homosexuals have entered medicine, they have encountered barriers because of their gender, race, class, age, or sexual orientation; many face obstacles because of more than one factor. They have sought personal coping mechanisms and strategies to change the structure of medicine, with its assumed norm of a white heterosexual male as the physician. In the process of attempting to alter the structures suited to the old norm, they sought to accommodate the lifestyles of more diverse individuals in order to allow them to become physicians. They fought for flexibility in curriculum, extended clerkships and residencies, reduction in overnight call, parental leave, and access to specialties within the training context. As they began to practice medicine, they struggled to obtain leadership positions on faculties, in hospitals and clinics, and on boards and committees to permit policy changes within the traditional white male hierarchy of the profession. While struggling for credibility and accommodation within the profession, these same individuals have had to struggle with allied health professionals and consumers in an attempt to change their perceptions and expectations about the white, rich, married male norm for a physician.

STATISTICS

Although in 1992–93 women constitute 41.6 percent of new entrants to medical schools nationally (Section for Student Services, 1992), they represent the base of a pyramid with steep sides in terms of the medical hierarchy. At each level of training and career advancement, women become a smaller percentage of the overall proportion of physicians.

In 1992 women earned 5,550/15,365, or 36.1 percent, of the M.D.'s (percentage calculated from Section for Student Services, 1992, p. 11). This percentage is significant compared to two decades ago, when women earned only 8.4 percent of the M.D.'s in 1970 (Bickel and Quinnie, 1992, Table 1). It takes considerably longer for the percentage increases of women in medical school to be translated into significant increases in the total population of physicians. In 1990 women constituted 104,194 of 615,421, or 17 percent, of all physicians (Bickel and Quinnie, 1992, Table 7).

In 1977 more than one-third of the specialties within medicine had no women residents; by 1985 women had entered all the major specialties (Altekruse and McDermott, 1988). However, in 1990, 53.3 percent of all women residents clustered in the three traditional specialties for women physicians: internal medicine (28.0 percent), pediatrics (15.1 percent), and psychiatry (10.2 percent) (data calculated from Bickel and Quinnie, 1992, Table 4). Almost 60 percent (61,526 of 104,194, or 59.0 percent) of all women physicians are grouped in the five following specialties, in rank order by size: internal medicine, pediatrics, general and family practice, psychiatry, and obstetrics/gynecology (data calculated from Bickel and Quinnie, 1992, Table 7).

Eighty-three percent of women physicians currently engage in patient care. For 47 percent this patient care is office-based. For 36 percent it is hospital-based; more than two-thirds of hospital-based physicians are residents (24 percent) or clinical fellows (2 percent). The other 17 percent of women physicians report other professional activity (7 percent) or inactive/not classified/no address (10 percent) as their primary activity (Bickel and Quinnie, 1992, Table 7).

The statistics on women in academic medicine serve as an important touchstone for gauging the status of women physicians in the overall profession. First, academic medicine includes both basic science and clinical faculty. Second, women in academic medicine serve as the first and most accessible role models for women medical students. Third, the hierarchy of academia, including ranks within the professoriate as well as administrative ranks such as department chair and dean, provide a means for gauging women's rising status within the profession.

A comparison of women faculty by department in 1975 and 1992 reveals that in all departments, both basic sciences and clinical, the percentage of women has increased on average: from 13.5 percent to 20.4 percent in the basic science departments, and from 14.6 percent to 22.8 percent in the clinical departments (Bickel and Quinnie, 1992, Table 5). Two-thirds of women in academic medicine occupy junior ranks within the professoriate. Specifically, 50.2 percent are assistant professors, 16.2 percent are instructors, and 3.4 percent hold other ranks. Only 9.5 percent of women are full professors, while 19.7 percent are associate professors (Bickel and Quinnie, 1992, Figure 1).

In contrast, more than half of men faculty hold the rank of full (31.5 percent) or associate professor (25.4 percent); only 34.5 percent, 6.6 percent, and 1 percent hold the respective ranks of assistant professor, instructor, or other (Bickel and Quinnie, 1992, Figure 1).

Of the women faculty, 78 percent (11,955) identify as white, 9.1 percent (1,393) as Asian, 3.7 percent (574) as Black, 2.9 percent (455) as Hispanic, 0.1 percent (19) as Native American, and 6.1 percent (937) as unknown ethnicity (calculated from Bickel and Quinnie, 1992, Figure 3). In 1990 only 16 percent (1,687) of 10,522 white women faculty were tenured. Sixteen and seven-tenths percent (1,760) were on tenure track; the majority (67.3 percent) were not on track (34.1 percent, or 3,583), not available (3.6 percent, or 381), or missing (29.6 percent, or 3,111) (Sherman, Johnson, and Whiting, 1990, Table 11B, p. 26). Only 12 percent (148) of the 1,237 Asian women faculty were tenured; 15.2 percent (188) were on tenure track. An even greater majority (72.8 percent) were not on track (38.9 percent, or 481), not available (2.3 percent, or 29), or missing (31.6 percent, or 391). Of the 459 Black women faculty, 11.1 percent (51) were tenured; 13.3 percent (61) were on tenure track. More than 75 percent were not on track (33.8 percent, or 155), not available (6.8 percent, or 31), or missing (35.1 percent, or 161). Of the 378 Hispanic women faculty, only 12.7 percent (or 48) were tenured; 14.3 percent (54) were on tenure track. The majority (276) were not on track (33.0 percent, or 125), not available (3.4 percent, or 13), or missing (36.5 percent or 138). Of the 17 Native American women faculty, 11.8 percent (2) were tenured; 5.9 percent (1) were on tenure track. More than four-fifths (82.4 percent, or 14) were not on track (41.2 percent, or 7) or missing (41.2 percent, or 7); none was listed as not available (calculated from Sherman, Johnson, and Whiting, 1990, Table 11B, p. 26).

These data suggest that although women now constitute 22.3 percent (15,333/68,821) of medical school faculty, they occupy the lower, least powerful ranks within the faculty. Relatively few have the security of tenure, and only 1,463 of 68,821 (2.1 percent) of all women faculty hold the rank of full professor (calculated from Bickel and Quinnie, 1992, Figure 1 and Table 5).

Few women faculty have the protection and prestigious status to hold the powerful theoretical and decision-making positions within the profession. In 1991–92, of the 90 women (42 in basic sciences, 45 in clinical sciences, 3 in interdisciplinary) chairing academic departments, 13 served only as acting or interim chair (Bickel and Quinnie, 1992, Table 6). Only 1 school of medicine out of 126 (0.7 percent) currently has a woman dean, Dr. Nancy Gary at Uniformed Services University of the Health Sciences, F. Edward Herbert School of Medicine (Bickel, 1992). However, 14.7 percent (414) of associate deans and 25.2 percent (102) of assistant deans in schools of medicine throughout the United States are women (Bickel and Quinnie, 1992, Table 8). These 1991–92 figures do represent considerable gains from 1975–76, when 0 percent, 3.4 percent, and 11.7 percent represented the respective percentages of women deans, associate deans, and assistant deans.

Achieving full rank and positions of leadership at the home university, hospital, or institute typically constitutes the first step toward a national leadership position. The dearth of women holding ranks such as department chair, dean, chief of staff, or head of the laboratory or institute translates into even smaller numbers of women on national boards, certification bodies, chairs of study sections for research panels, heads of national institutes, and presidents of state and national professional organizations.

The current leadership of American medicine fails to reflect the diversity of the changing medical profession and is even less reflective of the general population with regard to race, class, and sexual orientation, as well as gender. The continuing predominance of white, middle- to upper-class, heterosexual males in the leadership of American medicine complicates medical school and residency for the increasing numbers of students who deviate from the norm by at least one factor.

OBSTACLES ENCOUNTERED DURING MEDICAL TRAINING

The dramatic change in the gender composition of medical students during the past two decades and the initiatives to increase racial diversity have revealed a variety of obstacles students encounter as they struggle with schedules, institutions, and expectations of patients, faculty, and hospital staff geared toward a white, male medical student (Grant, 1988; Bickel, 1990; Knight, 1981; Ehrhardt and Sandler, 1990; Altekruse and McDermott, 1988). Most institutionalized forms of discrimination, such as admissions quotas based on gender or race, have been eliminated, since they became illegal with the passage of Title VII of the Civil Rights Act of 1964 and Title IX in 1972. Institutions have been less successful, however, in eradicating the kinds of blatant, subtle, and covert discrimination based on gender and race which students encounter frequently in admissions interviews, daily classroom and clinical interactions, channeling toward particular specialties, and schedules for completion of medical training.

All students enter medical school with more than twenty years of background training and socialization in American education and society. They have been subjected to socialization and sex-role stereotyping messages from parents, teachers, and the media which reinforce the image of the scientist and physician as a white male. A classic study (Chambers, 1983) recently repeated with students from a variety of backgrounds revealed that when asked to draw a scientist, only 28 out of 4,807 kindergarten students drew a picture of a female scientist; no little boys did so. This study, coupled with numerous others (e.g., National Science Foundation, 1992; Vetter, 1988) documenting that the percentage of women and people of color in science courses decreases from high school throughout college, makes students aware that medicine is a nontraditional career for men of color and all women (Ehrhardt and Sandler, 1990). Often challenged by families, peers, and communities about whether their decision to become a physician is realistic or "appropriate," men of color and women may question that decision when they encounter overt, subtle, or covert barriers during the demanding training in medical school.

In 1973 Mary Howell, using the pseudonym Margaret Campbell, wrote the book *Why Would a Girl Go into Medicine?* The title reveals a question from admissions committees, faculty, and patients that women seeking careers in medicine frequently had to answer. It exemplifies one of the types of discrimination outlined in that now-classic work.

Campbell (1973) defined behaviors such as baiting, belittling, hostility, and backlashing as overt discrimination. Baiting includes comments such as "Because of you a man probably went into chiropractic school" (Campbell, 1973, p. 23), intended to annoy or anger the women to whom they are addressed. The largest number of overtly discriminatory comments fall into the category of belittling remarks, such as "A woman doesn't belong in the OR except as a nurse," made by the chief of obstetrics-gynecology (p. 25). Hostile and backlash comments such as "Let her do it herself [lifting a heavy patient to examine the chest], she's liberated" (p. 29) appear to be undisguised and open expressions of free-floating anger against women.

Campbell included ostracizing, forgetting, spotlighting, stereotyping, and male prurience as subtle discrimination. Women medical students may be excluded from informal discussions over a beer after grand rounds (forgotten) or have their questions answered in a simplistic and condescending fashion (ostracism). In contrast, women may also endure having all questions regarding material on female sexuality addressed to them (spotlighting) and assumptions that certain behaviors and specialties such as pediatrics are more suitable for them because they are women (stereotyping). Pictures depicting female sexual practices, habits, and preferences such as "cheesecake" slides interspersed in anatomy lectures and remarks such as "The only significant difference between a woman and a cow is that a cow has more spigots" (Campbell, 1973, p. 41), made by a lecturer, represent male prurience exhibited in the medical classroom. These remarks and behaviors have a chilling effect on the classroom and clinical environment for women medical students. They also convey to male students that treating women colleagues and patients in this discriminatory fashion is not only tolerated but appropriate.

More recent studies (Grant, 1988) reveal that discrimination that might be labeled as fitting into each of these categories still exists in medical schools. For example, a study of first-year medical students at the Medical College of Ohio (Marquat, Franco, and Carroll, 1989) demonstrated that women were asked three times more often than men about their plans regarding marriage and children. This issue appears to persist even after success in medical school. During their interviews for residency programs, women students were asked more frequently than men about the stability of their personal relationships and their intention to have children (Association of American Medical Colleges, 1989). These interview questions exemplify a type of overt discrimination which Title IX made illegal in most cases. (Note: Such questions can be asked as long as they are asked of both men and women equally.)

Although discussed in *Why Would a Girl Go into Medicine?* sexual harassment has received more attention recently both from the general public and in schools of medicine. The Clarence Thomas hearings, the Navy Tailhook scandal, and the charges made by female employees of the Veterans Administration reported in *USA Today*, which later prompted Congressional hearings (Castenada, 1993), have sensitized the public to the existence of sexual harassment in the workplace, including the medical setting. Sexual harassment involves

> a specific form of gender discrimination characterized by unwelcome sexual advances, requests for sexual favors, and other verbal and physical conduct of a sexual nature where: submission to such conduct is made, either explicitly or implicitly, a condition of an individual's training or professional position and the conduct has the purpose or effect of unreasonably interfering with an individual's work or academic performance or of creating an intimidating, hostile or offensive work environment. (Lenhart and Evans, 1991, p. 77)

A study of students at ten medical schools (Ehrhardt and Sandler, 1990) revealed that 28.9 percent of women respondents had experienced sexual advances, 61.5 percent had endured sexist slurs, and 25.7 percent complained of sexist teaching materials. The structure of medical training is such that students are vulnerable to sexual harassment from a number of sources in a variety of settings. One study reports that approximately 33 percent of women experienced sexual harassment from a person in a position of authority; 46 percent experienced it from peers (Commission on Women's Issues, 1987). Other data suggest (Ehrhardt and Sandler, 1990) that women are most likely to experience sexual harassment or discrimination from clinical faculty members (two-thirds at least once). More than 60 percent of women named residents as the second most frequent source. Patients serve as another harassment source, with one-quarter of 1,120 female residents in one study (Dickstein and Botchelor, 1989) complaining of sexual come-ons by patients.

Sexual harassment does more than provide a dispiriting experience for women medical students and residents. It translates into negative models for behavior toward all women, including women patients and colleagues. When male medical students observe clinical faculty or residents harassing female students, they may model this behavior and begin to harass their female peers. It is not difficult to imagine how much more acceptable they may find it to harass women who are patients, over whom they have more power, than peers, who are their equals.

Incidents of sexual harassment, depending upon their severity and frequency, when combined with other barriers faced by women in medical education help to explain the data suggesting that women medical students, like women in other fields, consult with mental health services more frequently than do their male peers (Kris, 1985). Women report more role conflict, less familial support, fear of loss of relationships with families and partners, financial strain, and dread of public competition with men (Kris, 1985) than do men students. The term "microinequity" is often used to describe aspects of the work environment that cannot be addressed by legal means but that interfere with a person's growth and progress (Rowe, 1990). Bickel and Quinnie (1993) define the range of microinequities from unconscious slights to deliberate exploitation:

> *unconscious slights:* having negative presumptions made about one's professional capabilities or dedication, being left out of networks of peers, being referred to by one's first name when all the men are addressing one another as "doctor."

> *invisibility:* having one's suggestions be attributed to a man.

> *conscious slights:* the chief's knowingly scheduling important meetings at a time when a woman committee member cannot attend; a program head's publicly stating that a resident's pregnancy is an act of disservice to the department.

> *exploitation:* disproportionately assigning women teaching and clinical work; paying women lower salaries. (P. 21)

In 1992, the Accreditation Council for Graduate Medical Education voted that in order to receive accreditation, sponsoring institutions must provide residents with policies and procedures to address complaints of sexual harassment and exploitation (Bickel and Quinnie, 1993).

Both male and female students report stress from interpersonal conflicts with faculty, residents, peers, and nurses, particularly during clinical training. Spiegel, Smolen, and Hopfensperger (1987) report that women are more bothered than men by conflicts with medical school authorities, including nurses and peers, but that unlike men, they tend to react by increasing their efforts to succeed.

Additional sources of stress borne disproportionately by women medical students include inadequate pregnancy and parental leave, as well as provision for child care during medical education. Recent studies (Sinal, Weavil, and Camp, 1988; Sayres et al., 1986) show that most women in medicine plan their pregnancies and elect to have children during their residencies. A 1983 study (American Medical Association, 1984) of 1,364 women physicians found that about two-thirds of the respondents had children. Half had their first child during training; one-quarter had a second child during training. Finding that most institutions and programs had no formal policies, in December 1991 the AMA House of Delegates adopted recommendations encouraging medical specialty boards, residency programs, medical schools, and medical groups to develop written parental leave policies (Association of American Medical Colleges, 1992).

After the birth of a child, women in medicine face problems such as extended hours, rotating shifts, and special emergencies in addition to the typical child-care problems faced by all working women. Although a recent study (1990) showed that more than half of all teaching hospitals do include child-care centers, almost half of the one in four residents with at least one child do not have such facilities available to them (Dickstein and Botchelor, 1989).

STRATEGIES FOR IMPROVING THE SITUATION

The relatively rapid increase in the percentage of women in medical education during the past two decades means that many women have borne the brunt on an individual level of making changes in a system originally developed and used by white men. Many women found themselves in the position of being the test case for a particular issue or the pioneer in solving a problem for the institution or hospital as a whole. For example, 39 percent of respondents in one survey reported that they personally had known no other pregnant women physicians before they became pregnant. Most of these women were pioneers at their institution in negotiating their individual arrangements to accommodate pregnancy and early child care (Sinal, Weavil, and Camp, 1988).

As the number of women has increased, institutions have begun to develop formal policies and informal mechanisms to accommodate the diverse needs of women in medicine. As more women join medical school faculties and move through the ranks, they serve as role models for women students, while actively working for changes to make the medical school environment more female-friendly.

Pressure from women physicians, coupled with the growing evidence that medical schools were having problems in dealing with the increasing numbers of female students, led the Association of American Medical Colleges (AAMC) to establish the Office for Women in Medicine in 1976

(Bickel and Quinnie, 1993), currently Women's Programs under the Division of Institutional Planning and Development. This office provides programs at national meetings, holds administrative training seminars to advance women in medicine, publishes four newsletters each year and numerous other handbooks. It also encourages each medical school and teaching hospital to appoint a Women's Liaison Officer (WLO) to the AAMC. In addition to their role as an official contact for women between the AAMC and each institution, the credibility of AAMC has permitted some WLOs to serve as a focal point for organizing women and programs to address women's concerns on their individual campus.

On some campuses the WLO or another woman faculty member with administrative support has been successful in establishing an Office for Women in Medicine. For several years Harvard, Yale, SUNY-Buffalo, the University of Southern California, and Northeastern Ohio University College of Medicine have had such offices, which offer a variety of support services, counseling, and programs for women. Brown, Temple, and the Medical College of Virginia Commonwealth University have recently added an Office for Women in Medicine (Bickel and Quinnie, 1993). At McMaster University, innovations to include women's health in the curriculum have emerged from and been implemented by the Women's Health Office. A well-funded and active Office for Women in Medicine within a medical school symbolizes visible support for women in medicine to overcome remaining barriers within the institution.

The following profile of the Temple University School of Medicine Office of Women in Medicine published by the AAMC illustrates the activities typically undertaken by such an office.

Historically Temple has had an active AMWA chapter, a high percentage of women students and a number of activities such as career seminars and support groups. The decision to establish a formal Office of Women in Medicine (OWM) followed a series of open meetings to discuss interest in developing a more structured women's program. Advice was sought from established OWMs. Finally, women faculty and the associate dean for student affairs developed a proposal for presentation to the dean.

The major goals of Temple's OWM were articulated as follows: to provide administrative continuity to student groups, to assist in coordinating and planning personal and professional development programs, and to serve as a resource in the medical schools for issues concerning women. The dean supported the creation of the Office with limited funding but no dedicated space. The WLO, as associate dean for student affairs, became the director. The dean provided funding through the federal work-study program for two first-year medical students to help develop the OWM, which included creating a newsletter, gathering resources, planning programs, and studying how to ensure that language in the medical school became more gender-neutral (this work resulted in publication of a policy and a booklet "Guide to Non-sexist Language" that has proved very useful).

In the year since the OWM was formed, the dean appointed an ad hoc committee on the status of women faculty, providing these faculty a direct line of communication to the administration. Following a brief survey to all the faculty regarding perceptions of needs and priorities, that committee has initiated an annual review of faculty rank and salaries and planned a program on job negotiation and is now addressing parental leave policies. Recently the OWM began working with women students to become contacts and hosts for women applicants. Temple's Office of Development and Alumni Affairs now sends copies of the OWM newsletter to alumnae, and the Admissions Office publicizes OWM activities for recruitment purposes. (Bickel and Quinnie, 1993, p. 7)

THE IMPORTANCE OF HAVING A LARGE PERCENTAGE OF WOMEN IN MEDICINE

Today women enter medicine in greater numbers than ever before, marry in the same proportion as do their nondoctor sisters, and fulfill roles as both doctors and mothers (Battle, 1983). Typically as committed to medicine as their male peers, women are unwilling to ransom social and family experiences for the sake of practicing medicine. About half of the spouses of women in medicine are doctors, too (Myers, 1984). This pattern may help create incentives for greater institutional empathy for obligations related to pregnancy, child care, and other human endeavors.

Despite the barriers, discrimination, and long hours, women physicians report satisfaction with their chosen career. Many choose to join clinics and/or HMOs where regularly scheduled hours are more compatible with their family needs. Women physicians on the average receive lower incomes than their male colleagues; in 1988 women's income was 71 percent of men's (American Medical Association, 1991). Most women physicians are clustered in the specialties of general/internal medicine, psychiatry, pediatrics, and obstetrics/gynecology, where the average (male and female combined) salaries are $111,500, $127,600, $119,300, and $221,800 for each respective specialty. Seventy-one percent of those figures is substantially more than the salary of the average American woman (Beck et al., 1993). Career satisfaction and financial security provide two compelling reasons why increasing the numbers of women in medicine is good for women. Evidence suggests that increasing the numbers of women in medicine may also be good for medicine.

One motive that quantitatively and qualitatively differentiates women in medicine from male physicians has been the interest of women physicians in the community. The history of medicine reveals that they have promoted group-oriented preventive medicine and social hygiene activities, and have seen the link between medical problems, unhealthy living conditions, and behaviors of populations. Women physicians have tried to keep children well and have viewed older people in an interactive family context. Male physicians have tended to focus on autonomous practices or on leadership roles in institutional settings, on individual patients with acute medical and surgical problems, and on technological concerns even when the technology is primitive.

Regina Sanchez-Morantz (1988) tracked the historical record of U.S. physicians to detail the differing orientations of male and female health professionals. With women's roles channeled into community-focused educational activities and collaborative work with nurses, early women doctors practiced in community schools, orphanages, and what we now describe as voluntary health agencies. They initiated well-child clinics and mothers' milk banks, and urged humane laws to restrict child labor.

Women expended great effort to establish their own educational and clinical institutions. In the late 1800s, women medical doctors opened hospitals for women and for children. This gave them the opportunity to provide a full range of medical and surgical care not available to them in existing hospitals. Such stratification of the market was not a matter of choice; it was typically a last resort triggered by professional exclusion (Walsh, 1977).

The historical record clearly reflects the inclination of women in medicine—as both scientists and practitioners—to function as generalists, often across disciplinary lines. Women physicians predominantly select the comprehensive primary care areas of practice such as general internal medicine, preventive medicine, pediatrics, and family medicine (Altekruse and McDermott, 1988). They find it congenial to pursue multidisciplinary and often interinstitutional activities, although such ventures frequently evoke problems in attaining academic and professional recognition and reward.

Women's presence in the sciences, and in medicine in particular, surely counts among those multifactorial influences which are slowly reforming the patriarchal medical powerhouse and its "normal" way of doing business. The arrival of feminist thought and principles in medicine is beginning to be visible in the domains of research, education, and practice. Women in medicine have experienced circumscribed gains in recent years. However, the decentering of the white male physician as the norm for mainstream medicine will be aided by the outside pressures of women consumers as well as by women researchers, educators, or practitioners.

REFERENCES

Altekruse, Joan M., and McDermott, Suzanne W. 1988. Contemporary concerns of women in medicine. In Sue V. Rosser (ed.), *Feminism within the science and health care professions: Overcoming resistance.* Elmsford, N.Y.: Pergamon Press.

American Medical Association. 1991. *Women in medicine in America: In the mainstream.* Chicago: American Medical Association.

———. 1984. *Maternity leave for residents*, pp. 1–21. Chicago: American Medical Association.

Association of American Medical Colleges. 1989. *Facts and figures report.* Washington, D.C.: Association of American Medical Colleges.

————. 1992. Spotlight on parental leave policies. *Women in Medicine Update* 6, no. 3:2.

Battle, C. U. 1983. Working and motherhood: A view of today's realities. *Journal of the American Medical Women's Association* 38, no. 4:103–105.

Beck, Melinda; Hager, Mary; Rogers, Patrick; Miller, Susan; Rosenbery, Debra; and Snow, Katrin. 1993. Doctors under the knife. *Newsweek*, April 5, pp. 28–33.

Bickel, Janet. 1990. Women in medical school. In Sara E. Rix (ed.), *The American Woman 1990–1991: A status report.* New York: W. W. Norton and Co.

————. 1992. Gender differences among first-year medical students. *Women in Medicine Update* 6, no. 4:3–4.

Bickel, Janet, and Quinnie, Renee. 1992. *Women in medicine statistics.* Washington, D.C.: Association of American Medical Colleges.

————. 1993. *Buiding a stronger women's program: Enhancing the educational and professional environment.* Washington, D.C.: Association of American Medical Colleges.

Campbell, Margaret. 1973. *Why would a girl go into medicine? Medical education in the United States: A guide for women.* Old Westbury, N.Y.: Feminist Press.

Castenada, Carol. 1993. Report: Harassment at VA hospital. *USA Today,* January 18, p. A-1.

Chambers, D. W. 1983. Stereotypic images of the scientist: The Draw-a-Scientist Test. *Science Education* 67:255–265.

Commission on Women's Issues. 1987. *Sexual harassment survey.* University of Wisconsin–Madison: Center for Health Sciences.

Dickstein, Leah, and Botchelor, Allison. 1989. A national survey of women residents and stress. Paper presented at the annual meeting of the American Medical Women's Association, Los Angeles, October.

Ehrhardt, Julie, and Sandler, Bernice. 1990. *Rx for success: Improving the climate for women in medical schools and teaching hospitals.* Washington, D.C.: Project on the Status and Education of Women.

Grant, Linda. 1988. The gender climate of medical school: Perspectives of women and men students. *Journal of the American Medical Women's Association* 43 (July/August):176–198.

Jolly, Paul. 1993. Academic achievement and acceptance rates of underrepresented-minority applicants to medical school. *Academic Physician* (March):9–13.

Kahle, Jane. 1983. *The disadvantaged majority: Science education for women.* Burlington, N.C.: Carolina Biological Supply Co.

————. 1985. *Women in science.* Philadelphia: Falmer Press.

Knight, James A. 1981. *Doctor-to-be: Coping with the trials and triumphs of medical school.* New York: Appleton-Century-Crofts.

Kris, Kathryn. 1985. Developmental strains of women medical students. *Journal of the American Medical Women's Association* 40 (September/October):145–148.

Lenhart, S., and Evans, C. 1991. Sexual harassment and gender discrimination: A primer for women physicians. *Journal of American Medical Women's Association* 46:77–82.

Marquat, J.; Franco, K.; and Carroll, B. 1989. Gender differences in medical student interviews. Presented at the Association of American Medical Colleges' 1988 conference. Reported in *AAMC Women in Medicine Update* 3 (Winter):3.

Myers, M. F. 1984. Overview: The female physician and her marriage. *American Journal of Psychiatry* 141, no. 11:1386–1391.

National Science Foundation. 1992. *Women and minorities in science and engineering.* Washington, D.C.: Author.

Rowe, Mary. 1990. Barriers to equality: The power of subtle discrimination to maintain unequal opportunity. *The Employee Responsibilities and Rights Journal* 3:153–163.

Sanchez-Morantz, Regina M. 1988. *Sympathy and science.* New York: Oxford University Press.

Sayres, Maureen, et al. 1986. Pregnancy during residency. *New England Journal of Medicine* 314 (February 13):418–423.

Section for Student Services. 1992. In Janet Bickel and Renee Quinnie (eds.), *Women in medicine statistics.* Washington, D.C.: Association of American Colleges.

Sherman, Elizabeth A.; Johnson, David P.; and Whiting, Brooke E. 1990. *Participation of women and minorities on US medical school faculties 1980–1990: Faculty roster system.* Washington, D.C.: Association of American Medical Colleges.

Sinal, Sara; Weavil, Patricia; and Camp, Martha. 1988. Survey of women physicians on issues relating to pregnancy during a medical career. *Journal of Medical Education* (July) 63:531–538.

Spiegel, David; Smolen, Robert; and Hopfensperger, Kathryn. 1987. Interpersonal stress in medical education: Correlates for men and women students. *Journal of the American Medical Women's Association* 42 (January/February):19–21.

Thomas, Valerie. 1989. Black women engineers and technologists. *Sage* 6, no. 2:24–32.

Vetter, Betty. 1988. Where are the women in the physical sciences? In Sue V. Rosser (ed.), *Feminism within the science and health care professions: Overcoming resistance.* New York: Pergamon Press.

Walsh, Mary Roth. 1977. *Doctors wanted: No women need apply—Sexual barriers in the medical profession, 1837–75.* New Haven, Conn.: Yale University Press.

CHAPTER ELEVEN

Women's Ways of Knowing

Changing Teaching Techniques and Evaluation

Health care in the United States currently faces a state of crisis, transition, and reform. Costs have escalated dramatically during the last two decades. The total health care tab is currently $912 billion per year (Beck et al., 1993). It is estimated that the cost of health care jumped by approximately 10 percent in 1992. Fee-for-service costs increased by 14.2 percent, while health maintenance organization (HMO) costs increased an average of 8.8 percent in 1992 (Morganthau and Murr, 1993). Yet some 37 million Americans have no health insurance. Despite the fact that physicians' fees account for only 20 percent of the $912 billion health care tab, critics hold physicians largely responsible for runaway costs (Beck et al., 1993).

Concurrent with the escalating costs, the health care profession has experienced a dramatic increase in physicians, with the number almost doubling between 1965 and 1990, from 298,000 to 586,000. The ratio of physicians for every 100,000 people has risen from 148 to 237 during the same time period (Altman and Rosenthal, 1990). Virtually all of the growth has occurred among practitioners of medical specialties rather than practitioners of general medicine. In 1992, 85 percent of medical school graduates specialized (Salholz et al., 1993). Currently less than 30 percent of United States practitioners are generalists, compared to approximately 50 percent in most other industrialized countries (Task Force on the Generalist Physician, 1992). In its policy statement on the generalist physician (1992), the Task Force on the Generalist Physician of the Association of American Medical Colleges suggests that the ratio of specialists to generalists will become further unbalanced unless immediate, drastic changes occur.

> Over the past several years, our country has witnessed a marked growth of highly focussed subspecialist practitioners over more broadly based generalists. Even more problematic, the resulting practitioner imbalance is worsening year-by-year as a consequence of an increasingly skewed distribution of specialty training being selected by medical students and residents before they enter practice. (P. 2)

The surplus of physicians in some specialties practicing in desirable locations has spawned advertising and cutthroat competition among them. A substantial average income differential exists between the general/family practice physician, who earns $111,500, and many specialists such as surgeons ($233,800), obstetricians/gynecologists ($221,800), and radiologists ($229,800) (American Medical Association, as quoted in Beck et al., 1993). While escalating health care costs, this differential encourages medical school graduates to specialize, especially at a time when the median debt owed by medical school seniors with student loans is $55,859 (American Medical Association, 1993).

In a technologically advanced, industrialized country such as the United States, vaccination and other public health measures and medical technology have eradicated many of the microorganisms and anatomical causes for early death and shortened life span. Lifestyle factors, primarily under the control of the health care consumer, and environmental factors, perceived as out of the control of anyone, contribute to the shortened life span caused by the modern killers—cancer, cardiovascular disease, and AIDS. The role of the physician and the health care system in general in curing these diseases is limited. Widely publicized malpractice suits demonstrating neglect, poor judgment, or incompetence have led to further undermining of physician authority and credibility.

ROLES OF PHYSICIANS AND CONSUMERS

It has become obvious that the health care system must be revamped if it is to function efficiently and economically to provide access to more of the population. In addition to the far-reaching changes proposed by the government through the president's health care reform task force, there must be a major change regarding the relative roles that physicians and patients are permitted or forced to assume in the health care system. It should be questioned whether the role of physician as all-knowing authority making decisions for an ignorant, passive patient was ever humane, effective, or appropriate. However, the government, insurance companies, and federal and private health maintenance organizations are forcing changes in those roles. Second or third opinions are now required before insurance companies will agree to pay for many procedures; the number of days of hospitalization for which a patient may be reimbursed is frequently prescribed for a particular procedure. Nationwide, 61 percent of all employers now offer HMO membership to their employees, and 40 million Americans receive medical care in 45 states from approximately 600 HMOs (Morganthau and Murr, 1993, p. 39).

Expectations for the public as health care consumers are also changing. The growth of specialization, clinics, and health maintenance organizations has left the patient in sole possession of the holistic, comprehensive picture of his/her health formerly held by the family doctor. The consumer is responsible for knowing that some elective procedures may never be covered by insurance, and others will be covered only after "asking a nurse" or obtaining a second or third opinion. It has been hinted that insurance payments may soon be limited or prohibited for conditions such as emphysema, liver transplants, and skin cancer when they are proven to be caused by self-destructive behaviors such as smoking, drinking, and excessive tanning.

The changing health care system is forcing both physicians and health care consumers to change. The roles of physician as authority and patient as ignorant, unquestioning consumer are no longer viable. The need is for collaboration between a physician using his/her expert advice and train- ing, and a patient who is well educated in basic health and knowledgeable about the health care system to make responsible, informed decisions about his/her health. This could and should be the role of the generalist physician.

ROLE OF THE EDUCATIONAL SYSTEM

Unfortunately, our current educational system is not training either the physician or the public to undertake these new roles. Although the American Medical Association (AMA) and the medical schools recognize that the health care system is changing and that the authority of the physician has decreased (Bloom, 1988), most medical school curricula (and certainly those under which currently practicing physicians were trained) were modeled on the Flexner Report of 1910 (Flexner, 1910). This influ- ential report espoused a medical training model involving two years of basic science education (M-I and M-II) in the classroom and laboratory followed by two years of clinical education (M-III and M-IV) in inpatient hospital and outpatient clinic settings to produce a physician who is an autonomous separate authority (Bloom, 1988).

In 1932, Dr. Willard Rappeleye directed a review of all aspects of medical students' education for the AAMC; in the final report, numerous areas for improvement were outlined (Rappeleye, 1932). Although AAMC and professional scholars have continued to evaluate medical education and suggest improvements, the basic structure of medical education has changed little since that time.

> Since 1932, the AAMC and others have issued numerous studies, especially three important reports published in the 1980s, that reconfirmed and reiter- ated the 1932 Commission on Medical Education's findings and recommen- dations. These reports, plus the writings of several distinguished medical educators, show that during the 60 years following the 1932 report, some medical schools implemented some of the recommendations. But most re- sisted change, and the education of medical students in the late 1980s was, for the most part, little changed from that in the 1920s. (ACME-TRI, 1992)

Although some medical schools, such as Harvard's New Pathway Program, focus on the doctor-patient relationship beginning in the first two years, most still rely heavily on textbook learning (Dolan, Gwynne, and Simpson, 1989). The general education received by most laypersons in America is particularly deficient in information in basic science (Koshland, 1988) and health, thus perpetuating the ignorance and intimidation of the public and crippling its ability to deal with the new expectations of the evolving health care system.

In defense of the educational system, it should be pointed out that these changes in role expectations and in health care have occurred very rapidly. "Doctors who finished training as late as 1980 look at the field of medicine today and say they do not recognize the landscape" (Altman and Rosenthal, 1990). Less than a decade ago, health care consumers were encouraged to accept that the physician-as-authority model provided them with the best health care in the world (Ebert, 1986), just as the public accepted that the United States was the world leader in science and technology.

The public in the United States have begun to recognize that now is the time to improve their knowledge of science and technology so that they can continue to enjoy a high standard of living in an increasingly technological global economy; they are also recognizing that it is time to improve their knowledge of health and the health care system to enjoy a better quality of life. However, the move from recognition that there is a problem to actions that will provide solutions to these educational difficulties under new health care reform must occur rapidly. Are there any new models emerging from other fields that might aid both physicians and the public in grasping the educational position of each group and easing the transition to different roles?

WOMEN'S WAYS OF KNOWING

In 1986 the book *Women's Ways of Knowing*, written by Mary Field Belenky, Blythe McVicker Clinchy, Nancy Rule Goldberger, and Jill Mattuck Tarule, was published. Some had looked forward to the book for several years, having had their interest piqued by reports at national meetings about the research and tidbits gleaned from colleagues at the institutions where the research was taking place. Everyone sensed that this book and the research upon which it was based would have an impact on the academy.

That impact has been felt in numerous and diverse ways on campuses across the nation. Almost immediately, large numbers of women heralded it as an accurate chronicle of their experience with teaching and learning. It became required reading for all faculty on some campuses. Almost as quickly, critics emerged to question the methods, sample size, and extent to which the data might be generalized. Some women said this does not represent their experience; some men wondered why it was called *Women's Ways of Knowing* when it seems to reflect the way they know too.

Based upon their research, Belenky et al. examined *Women's Ways of Knowing* and described "five different perspectives from which women view reality and draw conclusions about truth, knowledge, and authority" (1973, p. 3):

> *silence,* a position in which women experience themselves as mindless and voiceless and subject to the whims of external authority; *received knowledge,* a perspective from which women conceive of themselves as capable of receiving, even reproducing, knowledge from the all-knowing external authorities but not capable of creating knowledge on their own; *subjective knowledge,* a perspective from which truth and knowledge are conceived of as personal, private, and subjectively known or intuited; *procedural knowledge,* a position in which women are invested in learning and applying objective procedures for obtaining and communicating knowledge; and *constructed knowledge,* a position in which women view all knowledge as contextual, experience themselves as creators of knowledge, and value both subjective and objective strategies for knowing. (P. 15)

They also distinguish two types of procedural knowing—separate and connected: "When we speak of separate and connected-knowing, we refer not to any sort of relationship between the self and another person but to relationships between knowers and the objects (or subjects) of knowing (which may or may not be persons)" (p. 102). Does the work of Belenky et al. offer any insights that might be helpful to the public and health care practitioners as we struggle for better health care and access for all, while keeping down spiraling costs?

Silence. In terms of knowing science and medicine, the majority of American health consumers, both male and female, fall under the first three perspectives on knowledge described by Belenky et al.: silent, received, and subjective knowers. Between 45 and 50 percent of people (Pion and Lipsey, 1981) think that science and technology have caused some of our problems. A substantial proportion of the population is overwhelmed by medicine and its methods and feels powerless in the face of scientific knowledge. For example, an Office of Technology Assessment survey in 1987 revealed that only 16 percent of the U.S. population rate their own basic understanding of science and technology as very good; 28 percent rate their understanding of science and technology as poor. The jargon of science and medicine may have been used to keep them in their place and make them fear questioning anything they hear that is scientific. The extent to which most students, regardless of grades, attempt to avoid science courses represents their silence toward and fear of science. The extent to which a substantial percentage of patients refuse to ask questions or reveal symptoms that may be causing them pain to a physician or other health care professional is a sign of their intimidation and silence before the health care system.

Received knowledge. Another considerable proportion of individuals, both male and female, appear to be received knowers. They accept without question and may repeat the information provided by the latest scientific and medical research findings presented by the scientist or surrogate authority for the scientist. Received knowers may change their life habits (what they eat, medications they give their children, the level of exercise they strive to achieve) without question, depending upon the latest research findings reported on the evening news. They may be overly compliant with a physician's instructions. They will continue with medication long after allergic reactions or other adverse side effects become evident. They may request new medications or change their habits based on the latest research findings popularized by the media even if the findings are not relevant to them. They do not have confidence in their own common sense or possess the knowledge to resolve conflicting information and data. Under the model of physician as authority, health care consumers in this group were perceived as ideal patients.

Subjective knowledge. Subjective knowers distrust and may even reject science and medicine and their methods and findings. No one really knows what percentage of the American population, both male and female, might fall into this camp. However, 29 percent of the population rate themselves as rather uninterested (11 percent) or not interested at all (18 percent) in scientific and technological matters (Office of Technology Assessment, 1987). Eighty-one percent of 755 people questioned in a Gallup poll for *Newsweek* in 1993 said that doctors charge too much. Forty-six percent said that doctors "keep patients waiting too long" (Beck et al., 1993). A 1989 poll also found that 26 percent of Americans say that they respect doctors less now than they did ten years ago. The most frequently cited reasons were that doctors were "in it for the money" or lacked concern for their patients. Seventeen percent think doctors do a poor job at keeping up with the latest medical knowledge. Thirty-five percent think they rate poorly in diagnosing patients correctly (Dolan, Gwynne, and Simpson, 1989).

Some patients, because of their distrust, may request tests and technologies that are inappropriate. Dr. Stephen Brenner, an internist in private practice in New Haven, Connecticut, said he is often pressured by patients who demand unnecessary tests and procedures. One way that HMO-managed care holds down costs is by limiting the rights of patients to request specific treatments. Dr. Terry Napal of the Greater Valley Medical Group in Los Angeles stated, "'When I was in private practice in Florida, we had all these affluent geriatric patients who'd come in and say they wanted an MRI because their friend had one. . . .' 'A lot of times, we gave it to them, even though it was breaking the system.' HMOs don't—or at least shouldn't—let that happen" (Morganthau and Murr, 1993, p. 39). Given the status and authority that medicine and physicians hold in our society and the popularity of quick cures, it appears that even a larger percentage of people in fact do not rely on medical knowledge and the health care system but refuse publicly to admit this rejection in favor of reliance on internal authority.

Procedural knowledge. According to Belenky et al. (1986), the scientific method, with its emphasis on subjectivity and distance between observer and object of study, is an example of separate, procedural knowing. As the data collected for *Women's Ways of Knowing* suggest, most college curricula and professors strive for their students to obtain the critical thinking skills, logical reasoning, and abstract analysis that characterize separate, procedural knowing.

Medicine as it is taught and practiced in the United States today exemplifies this type of knowing. Most pre-medical students, although encouraged to pursue majors in the humanities and social sciences, in fact major in one of the traditional sciences—usually biology, chemistry, or biochemistry. Considerable research (Keller, 1985) applying feminist theories from psychology such as the work of Chodorow (1978) and Gilligan (1982) suggests that individuals who value autonomy, distance, and masculinity will feel comfortable in science and succeed in science courses. Feminist philosophers, historians, and scientists have considered the extent to which the mechanistic, objective approach to science that supplanted the hermetic, organic approach in the seventeenth century might be synonymous with a masculine world view (Keller, 1985; Merchant, 1979).

Not all individuals interested in careers in medicine fit these descriptors, nor was the masculinity of science the major barrier that prevented women from entering medicine until the last two decades. However, individuals who are not adept at learning through the separate, procedural way in which science courses are taught are unlikely to be successful applicants to medical school. The separate, procedural approach is further emphasized in the first two years of medical school, which are devoted to basic science. The voluminous amount of information delivered in a compressed time frame, coupled with competitive and distancing methods used in teaching most M-I and M-II courses, vastly surpassed the extent to which separate procedural knowledge is emphasized on the undergraduate level.

The 1932 review of the medical curriculum pointed toward overcrowding and rigidity in the curriculum: "The almost frantic attempt to put into the medical course teaching all phases of scientific and medical knowledge, and the tenacity with which traditional features of teaching are retained have been responsible for great rigidity, overcrowding, and a lack of proper balance in the training" (Rappeleye, 1932).

Even after the clinical years, most physicians emerge prepared to assume the role of physician as authority. They themselves may be capable of becoming connected or constructed knowers, although recent concern over excessive compartmentalization resulting in separation of basic science from clinical knowledge in board examinations suggests that many physicians have not yet reached that stage at the end of their medical training. The 1932 review indicates that this is a problem that has plagued medical education for decades: "Too much of the clinical teaching is from the standpoint of the specialist and on rare diseases. Insufficient attention is given to the ordinary needs of most patients" (Rappeleye, 1932).

A 1984 report (Muller, 1984) called for an integrated, interdisciplinary approach to undergraduate medical education:

> Medical school deans should identify and designate an interdisciplinary and interdepartmental organization of faculty members to formulate a coherent and comprehensive educational program for medical students and to select the instructional and evaluation methods to be used. Drawing on the faculty resources of all departments, this group should have the responsibility and the authority to plan, implement and supervise an integrated program of general professional education. The educational plan should be subject to oversight and approval by the general faculty.

However, the ACME-TRI report (1992) *Educating Medical Students* found that only 20 of 84 responding schools had implemented this recommendation to some degree (all 126 medical schools were sent the survey). As a necessary strategy for change, this report again recommends "integrated and coordinated education programs for medical students" (p. 5).

Certainly little in their training prepares physicians to aid the public, who represent the first three stages of knowing, in becoming connected or constructed knowers. Rather, the current training of physicians to be separate, autonomous knowers and authority figures represents the antithesis of what is needed.

Constructed knowledge. Despite their training as separate, procedural knowers in the traditional courses and programs that prepare scientists to undertake scientific and medical research, some women Ph.D.'s and M.D.'s have demonstrated that they are connected knowers. Their basic research in health and medicine emphasizes connections that shape the definition and choice of problems studied, approaches used, and conclusions and applications drawn from the research.

Considerable attention (Wheeler, 1990) has recently been drawn to the failure of the National Institutes of Health (NIH) to include female research subjects and to study diseases of women. Women researchers have suggested that recognition of the importance of gender is crucial for the definition of the problem studied and the wording of the hypothesis. As Messing states: "Articulating the hypothesis is crucial to the scientific method. Research is done in order to find an answer to a specific question, and the way the question is posed often determines the way the research will be carried out and how the eventual data will be interpreted" (Messing, 1983, p. 78). Part of the focus on gender might be demonstrated in research topics of particular concern to women.

Women researchers have also urged broader definitions of what constitutes scientific research. Some types of research of importance to women have been defined as nonscience because of who undertook the research. Because science is considered a masculine pursuit in our culture (Harding, 1986; Keller, 1985), science performed by women is often defined as nonscience. H. Patricia Hynes (1984) documents the redefinition of Ellen Swallow Richards's experiments in water chemistry, toxicity, and food purity out of the science of chemistry and into home economics. Her work was considered unscientific because it was interdisciplinary research done by a woman.

In *For Her Own Good* Barbara Ehrenreich and Deirdre English (1978) explore the ways in which methods to aid birthing are considered to be science or nonscience depending upon who is practicing them. Midwifery is not usually considered a science because it is practiced by women, although obstetrics is a science because it is a medical field dominated by men.

Information growing out of women's personal experiences, which have formerly been ignored or understudied, may provide significant insights for researchers. In the area of health care, women have often reported (and accepted among themselves) experiences that could not be documented by scientific experiments or were not accepted as valid by the researchers of the day. Cases of toxic shock syndrome were reported by the women upon whom the Rely tampon was tested. The Procter and Gamble Company chose not to reveal these data until litigation ensued (Marwick, 1983).

In "A Case of Corporate Malpractice and the Dalkon Shield," Mark Dowie and Tracy Johnston (1977) document that many of the problems with the Dalkon Shield had been uncovered during the testing and early marketing phases of the development of the IUD (intrauterine device). The A. H. Robins Company and the developers of the shield chose to ignore that data. The company continued the coverup even when reports accumulated of severe complications and deaths from the Dalkon Shield due to problems similar to those reported during its development. Only legal action from women harmed by this device brought the initial test results to light and resulted in its removal from the market.

Not only have women researchers been willing to make connections with problems of significance for women's health and explore nontraditional topics growing out of women's experiences, but they have also been willing to investigate expanded approaches to solving the problems. Because the scope of problems explored by women tends to be broader, methods which cross disciplinary boundaries or include combinations of methods traditionally used in separate fields may provide more appropriate approaches.

The 1932 Rappeleye Commission Report called for medical education to include the context of the larger social and economic problems with which medicine deals:

Inasmuch as medical education is primarily concerned with the qualification and preparation of students to practice medicine, it is highly important that the training be permeated with an understanding of the larger social and economic problems and trends with which medicine must deal, and which are likely to influence the form and opportunities of practice in the future. (Rappeleye, 1932)

The ACME-TRI Report (1992) encourages faculty members to teach outside their disciplines.

Schools must create meaningful cross-disciplinary teaching opportunities to encourage faculty members to assume educational responsibilities beyond their specialized area of practice or research. Equally important, faculty members must participate in cross-disciplinary examinations of students. An example of a specific approach to achieve this is problem-based learning. Problem-based learning is a method of teaching around case problems in which the role of the faculty member is one of resource person rather than expert. This approach to teaching fosters interdisciplinary teaching and stimulates faculty members to become involved in teaching subjects outside their respective disciplines or specialties. (ACME-TRI, 1992)

Cross-disciplinary approaches would promote education of the generalist physician, encourage "connected" or "constructed" learning, and foster interdisciplinary approaches to research problems.

Some researchers have been more willing to use interactive methods which shorten the distance between the observer and the subject being studied. Elizabeth Fee (1983) provides an account of such interactive methods in her work on occupational health research in an Italian factory (see the chapter on methodologies).

In the conclusions drawn from the data, many women researchers have sought to make connections among multiple, interdependent, and related causes for effects rather than adopting hierarchical, reductionistic, and dualistic explanations. Bleier uses a particularly appropriate example to demonstrate the shortcomings of the nature/nurture dualism in the theory of fetal development:

Since we tend to take for granted (or ignore) the normal physiological milieu as an essential part of development, it is easier to recognize the influence of environmental milieu on genetic expression if we consider external environmental factors that affect fetal development in humans through their disruptive effects on the maternal milieu. The mother's diet, drug ingestion (for example, thalidomide, DES, alcohol), virus infections (such as herpes and German measles), stress, and other known factors may have serious effects on the physical characteristics of the developing fetus. In some way all of these environmental characteristics have the capacity to induce abnormalities in the environmental milieu of the fetus, and it is the interactions between genetic factors and disturbed internal environmental factors that result in altered fetal development. There is no way to tease apart genetic and environmental factors in human development or to know where genetic effects end and environmental ones begin; in fact, this is a meaningless way to view the problem since from conception the relationships between the gene's protein synthesizing activity and the fetus' maternal environment are interdependent. As Lappe has said, "Genes and environments do not simply 'add up' to produce a whole. The manner in which nature and nurture interact to cause biological organisms to flourish or decline is an extraordinarily complex problem." (Bleier, 1984, p. 43)

Many researchers have sought to exert, wherever possible, positive control over the practical use of their scientific discoveries with a consideration toward helping human beings.

Then we, as feminist scientists, in making explicit our own social values and beliefs where they are relevant to the science we practice, may wish to claim a feminist approach to scientific knowledge that in its language, methods, interpretations, and goals, acknowledges its commitments to particular human values and to the solution of particular human problems. This would not eliminate or censor basic scientific investigations done for the sake of knowledge itself, with no known practical, social application, but it would aim to eliminate research that leads to the exploitation and destruction of nature, the destruction of the human race and other species, and that justifies the oppression of people because of race, gender, class, sexuality, or nationality. (Bleier, 1984, p. 16)

Most of these examples from the work of women researchers emphasize connection in some way: connection with the practical uses for which the discovery will be used; a chosen connection with the object of study; connection with other related scientific problems; and, most important, connection between science and human beings.

Examination of the work of women researchers yields evidence that they are connected knowers. Because almost all of the examples discussed come from the work of successful scientists who obtained degrees from traditional institutions of higher education, most would be classified as constructed knowers. They have the ability to "view all knowledge as contextual, experience themselves as creators of knowledge, and value both subjective and objective strategies for knowing" (Belenky et al., 1986, p. 15). However, it appears that connected knowing on some level is an important step or aspect of the constructed knowledge for these women.

Who in the health care system can help the health care consumer make this transition to connected knowledge? How can the medical education of physicians be changed to move all physicians, particularly generalist physicians, from the stage of separate, procedural knowers through the stage of connected knowing to become constructed knowers?

Only if physicians themselves have reached the stage of constructed knowing will they be able to help their patients and the public understand what they need to know about their own health and health care. Since most patients fall into the categories of silent, received, and subjective knowers as health care consumers, they have not reached the stage of knowledge that enables them to cope effectively with the new role required of health care consumers in the changing health care system. Nurses and nurse practitioners have traditionally helped patients to mesh their needs with those of the health care system. The generalist physician must also be educated to help the consumer mediate the system.

> The system of managed care heavily depends on a gatekeeper, usually an internist or a family-care physician, . . . who can look the patient in the eye and credibly say, "You don't need that." This takes close familiarity with the patient's medical history and, above all, trust. (Morganthau and Murr, 1993, p. 39)

In its emphasis upon integrated, interdisciplinary medical education in which information in basic science courses and clinical training is presented in the context of social and economic issues, the ACME-TRI Report (1992) suggests curricular approaches to provide physicians with the information needed to become constructed knowers. Following upon the recommendation of the 1980s reports (1983, 1984), ACME-TRI stresses changes in procedures to evaluate medical students.

> We recommend that faculty review their educational goals to ascertain that both the content and methods of evaluation are compatible with these goals. To attain congruence a variety of testing techniques should be used: tests of problem-solving skills, in addition to factual recall; tests of noncognitive educational outcomes, such as proficiency in performing procedures, in addition to written tests addressing cognitive outcomes; tests, oral and written, that require students to generate original responses, rather than select responses from a given list. (Friedman and Purcell, 1983)

> Current examination techniques that rely principally on students' abilities to recall memorized information should be complemented by examinations that assess students' problem-solving and patient-evaluation skills. As faculty members become familiar with such examinations, they should gradually introduce them to replace multiple-choice testing, which is now the most common testing approach. . . .

> Schools need to recognize that the evaluation of students depends on more than the type of assessment technique or form used. The entire *system* of evaluation needs to be considered: How is information passed from one course to the next? Is there a student committee with oversight and timely information about students' progress through all four years of medical school? Is there a mechanism for assuring the student has met all established criteria and is able to begin a residency program upon graduation? (ACME-TRI, 1992, p. 25)

The ACME-TRI Report (1992) also reinforces the recommendation of the 1984 report that medical education foster self-directed learning and the acquisition of lifelong learning skills. The physician practicing in the twenty-first century must be able to stay current with the constant changes in medical practice. Much of the science and technology that form the basis for medical practice that students are taught in medical school, especially during the first and second years, has changed in important ways by the time they complete their residencies. The amount of information compressed into the four years of medical school cannot be memorized and later applied to the care of a human being. This concept is well stated in the following recommendation:

> To keep abreast of new scientific information and new technology, physicians continually need to acquire new knowledge and learn new skills. Therefore, a general professional education should prepare medical students to learn throughout their professional lives rather than simply mastering current information and techniques. Active, independent, self-directed learning requires among other qualities the ability to identify, formulate, and solve problems; to grasp and use basic concepts and principles, and to gather and assess data rigorously and critically. *General Professional Education of the Physician*, 1984. (ACME-TRI, 1992, p. 36)

Changing evaluation to reinforce synthesis and integration from a variety of types of information and sources provides a tool for becoming a constructed knower. Fostering self-directed learning and acquisitional skills for lifelong learning gives the physician an additional incentive for continuing to be a constructed knower.

As constructed knowers, generalist physicians will "view all knowledge as contextual, experience themselves as creators of knowledge, and value both subjective and objective strategies for knowing" (Belenky et al., 1986, p. 15). From that vantage point they can aid others, particularly patients, but also specialists, in connecting with each other and with knowledge about health and the health care system. In this crisis period that health care currently faces, generalist physicians, methods employed by some women researchers, and nurse practitioners and their knowledge are the vital connection that can provide the transition to better health care for all.

REFERENCES

ACME-TRI. 1992. *Educating Medical Students*. Washington, D.C.: Association of American Medical Colleges.

Altman, Lawrence K., and Rosenthal, Elisabeth. 1990. Changes in medicine bring pain to healing profession. *The New York Times*, February 18, pp. 1(A), 20–21(A).

Beck, Melinda; Hager, Mary; Rogers, Patrick; Miller, Suzann; Rosenberg, Debra; and Snow, Katrin. 1993. Doctors under the knife. *Newsweek*, April 5, pp. 28–33.

Belenky, Mary Field; Clinchy, Blythe McVicker; Goldberger, Nancy R.; and Tarule, Jill Mattuck. 1986. *Women's ways of knowing.* New York: Basic Books.

Bleier, Ruth. 1984. *Science and gender: A critique of biology and its theories on women.* Elmsford, N.Y.: Pergamon Press.

———. 1986. Introduction. In Ruth Bleier (ed.), *Feminist approaches to science,* p. 16. Elmsford, N.Y.: Pergamon Press.

Bloom, Samuel W. 1988. Structure and ideology in medical education: An analysis of resistance to change. *Journal of Health and Social Behavior* 29 (December):294–306.

Chodorow, Nancy. 1978. *The reproduction of mothering: Psychoanalysis and the sociology of gender.* Berkeley and Los Angeles: The University of California Press.

Dolan, Barbara; Gwynne, S. C.; and Simpson, Janice. 1989. Sick and tired. *Time,* July 31, pp. 48–53.

Dowie, Mark, and Johnston, Tracy. 1977. A case of corporate malpractice and the Dalkon Shield. In Claudia Dreifus (ed.), *Seizing our bodies,* pp. 86–104. New York: Vintage Books.

Ebert, Robert. 1986. Medical education at the peak of the era of experimental medicine. *Daedalus* 115:55–81.

Ehrenreich, Barbara, and English, Deirdre. 1978. *For her own good: 150 years of the experts' advice to women.* Garden City, N.Y.: Anchor Books.

Fee, Elizabeth. 1982. A feminist critique of scientific objectivity. *Science for the People* 14, no. 4:5–8, 30–33.

———. 1983. Women's nature and scientific objectivity. In Marian Lowe and Ruth Hubbard (eds.), *Woman's nature: Rationalizations of inequality,* p. 24. Elmsford, N.Y.: Pergamon Press.

Flexner, Abraham. 1910. *Medical education in the United States and Canada: A report to the Carnegie Foundation for the Advancement of Teaching.* New York: Carnegie Foundation. Reprint. New York: Arno, 1972.

Friedman, C. P., and Purcell, E. F. (eds.). 1983. *The new biology and medical education: Merging the biological, information, and cognitive sciences.* New York: Josiah H. Macy, Jr. Foundation.

Gilligan, Carol. 1982. *In a different voice: Psychological theory and women's development.* Cambridge, Mass.: Harvard University Press.

Harding, Sandra. 1986. *The science question in feminism.* Ithaca, N.Y.: Cornell University Press.

Hynes, H. Patricia. 1984. Women working: A field report. *Technology Review,* November/December, pp. 37–39, 41.

Keller, Evelyn Fox. 1985. *Reflections on gender and science.* New Haven and London: Yale University Press.

Kolata, Gina. 1990. Doctor-patient relationships take a turn for the worse. *Columbia (SC) State,* March 27, pp. 1(D), 7(D).

Koshland, Daniel. 1988. Women in science. *Science* 239 (March 17):4847.

Marwick, C. 1983. Holdup of toxic shock data ends during trial in Texas. *Journal of American Medical Association* 250, no. 4:3267–3269.

Merchant, Carolyn. 1979. *The death of nature: Women, ecology, and the scientific revolution.* San Francisco: Harper and Row.

Messing, Karen. 1983. The scientific mystique: Can a white lab coat guarantee purity in the search for knowledge about the nature of women? In Marian Lowe and Ruth Hubbard (eds.), *Woman's nature: Rationalizations of inequality.* Elmsford, N.Y.: Pergamon Press.

Morganthau, Tom, and Murr, Andrew. 1993. Inside the world of an HMO. *Newsweek,* April 5, pp. 34–40.

Muller, S. (Chairman). 1984. Physicians for the twenty-first century: Report of the Project Panel on the General Professional Education of the Physician and College Preparation for Medicine. *Journal of Medical Education* 59, no. 2.

Office of Technology Assessment. 1987. *New developments in biotechnology background paper: Public perceptions of biotechnology.* OTA-BP-BA-45. Washington, D.C.: Government Printing Office.

Pion, Georgine M., and Lipsey, Mark W. 1981. Public attitudes toward science and technology: What have the surveys told us? *Public Opinion Quarterly* 45.

Rappeleye, W. C. (Director). 1932. *Medical education: Final report of the Commission on Medical Education.* New York: Association of American Medical Colleges.

Salholz, Eloise; Beachy, Lucille; Wilson, D. J.; and Gordon, Jean. Future shock for med students. *Newsweek*, April 5, 1993, p. 31.

Task Force on the Generalist Physician. 1992. *Executive summary.* Washington, D.C.: Association of American Medical Colleges.

Wheeler, D. L. 1990. NIH to require researchers to include women in studies. *The Chronicle of Higher Education* 37, no. 3:32–33(A).

Conclusion

Modern medicine has failed to include women in substantive ways. The absence of large numbers of women holding theoretical and decision-making positions within the ranks of physicians and researchers has been reflected in research topics and protocols flawed by androcentric bias. The results of this biased research become translated into diagnoses and treatments which tend to be less appropriate for women, and in some extreme cases, such as angioplasty, result in death rates for women that are ten times higher than those for men who undergo the same procedure.

Each clinical specialty traces its roots to at least one of the basic sciences. The problems chosen for study, methods and approaches, and prevailing theories in the basic sciences often reflect a unique but lengthy history of embedded androcentrism. Each clinical specialty builds on its related basic science foundation, adding particular twists, including gender bias, to its own history of clinical research.

Androcentrism appears to take different forms, resulting in different effects in the various specialties. For example, androcentrism in AIDS research in the United States took the form of focus on the male only. Since susceptibility to AIDS was defined by groups—male homosexuals, IV drug users, and Haitian immigrants—rather than risk behaviors, women were excluded from the Centers for Disease Control (CDC) case definition for AIDS until 1993, testing for drugs effective against the virus, and studies of transmission of the disease. This male focus has resulted not only in women being the group in which AIDS is increasing most rapidly in the United States but also in a growing epidemic among the heterosexual population. In contrast, in psychiatric research and diagnosis, androcentrism has manifested itself somewhat differently. With the male life cycle and male psychology being used as the norm, events normal to the lives of most women are defined as disease syndromes or problematic conditions. Sex-role expectations about appropriate or disruptive behaviors based upon women's functioning within a family may lead to underdiagnosis of alcoholism and overdiagnosis of depression in women.

The specialty of obstetrics/gynecology illustrates yet a further dimension of androcentrism. Although research in obstetrics/gynecology uses females as experimental subjects and methods appropriate for the female body, the focus of research problems and practice is largely defined by women's health issues resulting from heterosexual sex—sexually transmitted diseases, contraception, infertility, pregnancy, childbirth, and menopause. Since obstetrics/gynecology has been designated as the specialty devoted to women's health, this definition through heterosexual sex leaves many women's health issues understudied and many women untreated. Indeed, the bias takes its toll not only on women, but also on men and children, who suffer from misunderstanding of AIDS risks and transmission and from failure to understand the impact of poor nutrition and poor health on individuals who bear the children of both genders.

Women of color, elderly women, and/or lesbians experience the effects of sexism combined with racism, ageism, and/or homophobia. Not only does each group have needs that distinguish it from the other groups, but each also has different relationships and maintains different distances from the mainstream clinical research. Given the difficulties with androcentrism and the problems with making research on women's health a national priority, it is not surprising that research on the health of these diverse groups of women is virtually nonexistent. Since an individual woman may simultaneously or eventually belong to one or all of these groups, research on the effects of age, race, and sexual orientation, as well as gender, must become an integral part of the research agenda for the health of women. Failure to distinguish and define needed research for each of these groups of women leaves them ignorant of their own health and disease and confounds research on diseases confined primarily to Caucasian heterosexually active women of reproductive age.

Some of the research and teaching techniques from the newly emerging fields of women's studies and ethnic studies may provide insights and may be used as models to make medical research and the medical curriculum more inclusive of all women and men of color. An exploration of different feminist theories reveals some methodologies that might have useful implications in examining issues in women's health. Models used to integrate women's studies and ethnic studies into traditional curricula suggest that a specialty in women's health would ensure the inclusion of women and women's health in all aspects of medicine.

Eliminating the barriers and the chilly climate for women in medicine is important not simply to increase the numbers and diversity in the pool of physicians. The small number of women physicians and researchers have demonstrated a particular interest in what is sorely needed as our nation faces its current health care crisis. The historical record clearly reflects the inclination of women in medicine—as both scientists and practitioners—to function as generalists, often across disciplinary lines. Women physicians predominantly select the comprehensive primary care areas of practice such as general internal medicine, preventive medicine, pediatrics, and family medicine. Women serve as the generalist physicians needed to help the health care consumer connect with the knowledge s/he must have regarding health and disease processes. Including interests and practice styles of women physicians and the research needs of all women in the health research agenda is crucial for the health of the nation, which depends on the health of its women.

Women and Health:
A Selected Bibliography

COMPILED BY FAYE A. CHADWELL

Abram, Ruth (ed.). 1985. *Send us a lady physician: Women doctors in America, 1835–1920.* New York: Norton.

ACT UP/New York Women and AIDS Book Group. 1990. *Women, AIDS, and activism.* Boston: South End Press.

AIDS among women to double by 2000. 1991. *Public Health Reports* 106 (March/April):216.

Allen, Deborah I. 1989. Women in medical specialty societies: An update. *JAMA* 262:3439–3443. Discussion, *JAMA* 263:2298.

AMA Data Source. 1989. *Women in medicine.* Chicago: American Medical Association.

Amaro, Hortensia, and Russo, Nancy F. 1987. Hispanic women and mental health: An overview of contemporary issues in research and practice. *Psychology of Women Quarterly* 11:393–407.

Anastos, K., and Marte, C. 1989. Women—The missing persons in the AIDS epidemic. *Health/PAC Bulletin* 6 (Winter):13.

Anderson, Ann, and McPherson, Anne (eds.). 1983. *Women's problems in general practice.* New York: Oxford University Press.

Anderson, Christopher. 1992. Women in research: NIH aims at "glass ceiling." *Nature* (March 5):6.

Andrist, Linda C. 1988. A feminist framework for graduate education in women's health. *Journal of Nursing Education* 27(2):66–70.

Apple, Rima (ed.). 1990. *Women, health, and medicine in America: A historical handbook.* New York: Garland.

Arber, Sara. 1990. Opening the "Black" box: Understanding inequalities in women's health. In P. Abbott and G. Payne (eds.), *New directions in the sociology of health,* pp. 37–56. Brighton: Falmer.

Arber, Sara, and Gilbert, G. Nigel. 1989. Transitions in caring: Gender, life course and the care of the elderly. In W. R. Bytheway (ed.), *Becoming and being old: Sociological approaches to later life,* pp. 72–92. London: Sage.

Armitage, Karen J.; Schneiderman, L. J.; and Bass, R. A. 1979. Response of physicians to medicial complaints in men and women. *JAMA* 241 (May 18):2186–2187.

Arnold, R. M.; Martin, S. C.; and Parker, R. M. 1988. Taking care of patients: Does it matter whether the physician is a woman? *Western Journal of Medicine* 149(6):729–733.

Ashley, Jo Ann. 1980. Power in structured misogyny: Implications for the politics of care. *Advances in Nursing Science* 2(3):3–22.

Banzhaf, Marion. 1990. *Women, AIDS and activism.* (Spanish edition *Mujeres, SIPA, and Activisimo.*) Boston: South End Press.

Baumgard, Alice. 1985. Women's health: Directions for the 80s. *Health Care for Women International* 6:267–276.

Beckwith, Barbara. 1985. Boston women's health book collective: Women empowering women. *Health Care for Women International* 10(1):1–9.

Beery, M. 1990. Women and HIV/AIDS. *Washington Nurse* 20 (November–December):27.

Bell, Nora K. 1989. Women and AIDS: Too little, too late? *Hypatia* 4 (Fall):3–22.

Bell, Susan. 1987. Changing ideas: The medicalization of menopause. *Social Science and Medicine* 24:535–542.

Bennett, Maisha. 1987. Afro-American women: Poverty and mental health—A social essay. *Women and Health* 12(3/4):213–228.

Bernstein, Barbara, and Kane, Robert. 1981. Physicians' attitudes toward female patients. *Medical Care* 19(6):600–608.

Beyene, Y. 1986. Cultural significance and physiological manifestations of menopause: A biocultural analysis. *Culture, Medicine, and Psychiatry* 10(1):47–71.

Bickel, Janet. 1988. Women in medical education: A status report. *New England Journal of Medicine* 310 (December 15):1579–1584. Discussion, 320 (May 18, 1989):1348–1350.

Bishop, Joan. 1992. Guidelines for a non-sexist (gender-sensitive) doctor-patient relationship. *Canadian Journal of Psychiatry* 37(1):62–65.

Bluestone, Naomi. 1985. A woman for a doctor. *Health* 17 (November):21–25.

Bobula, Joel D. 1980. Work patterns, practice characteristics, and income of male and female physicians. *Journal of Medical Education* 55:826–833.

Bonner, Thomas N. 1992. *To the ends of the earth: Women's search for education in medicine.* Cambridge, Mass.: Harvard University Press.

Boston Women's Health Book Collective. 1992. *The new our bodies, ourselves: Updated and expanded for the nineties.* New York: Simon and Schuster.

Boughn, Susan. 1991. A women's health course with a feminist perspective: Learning to care for and empower ourselves. *Nursing Health Care* 12(2):76–80.

Bowman, Marjorie, and Allen, Deborah I. 1990. *Stress and women physicians.* 2nd ed. New York: Springer-Verlag.

Bowman, Marjorie, and Gross, Marcy Lynn. 1986. Overview of research on women in medicine—Issues for public policymakers. *Public Health Reports* 101 (September/October):513–521.

Braithwaite, Ronald L., and Taylor, Sandra E. (eds.). 1992. *Health issues in the Black community.* San Francisco: Jossey-Bass.

Bunkle, Phillida, and Hughes, Beryl (eds.). 1988. *Second opinion: The politics of women's health in New Zealand.* Auckland, New Zealand: Oxford University Press.

Bureau of National Affairs. 1989. *Working women's health concerns: A gender at risk?* Washington, D.C.: Bureau of National Affairs.

Burke, Harry B. 1986. Female frosh fare fine. *JAMA* 256 (December 26):3348.

Burke, Harry B. 1991. Improving older women's health. *Geriatrics* 46 (November):15.

Butler, Robert N. 1991. Further estrogen studies need vigorous pursuit. *Geriatrics* 46 (April):15.

Byron, Peg. 1991. HIV—The national scandal. *Ms.* 1 (January/February):24–29.

Calhoun, Cheshire. 1988. Justice, care, and gender bias. *Journal of Philosophy* 85(9):451–463.

Campbell, Courtney. 1990. My fair lady (NIH and inclusion of women in medical research studies). *Hastings Center Report* 20 (September/October):3.

Campbell, Courtney. 1990. Women and AIDS. *Social Science and Medicine* 30(4):407–415.

Campbell, Margaret A. 1973. *Why would a girl go into medicine?* New York: Feminist Press.

Carmen, Elaine H.; Russo, N. F.; and Miller, J. B. 1981. Inequality and women's mental health: An overview. *American Journal of Psychiatry* 38(10):1319–1330.

Caserta, Joan. 1990. Women in the 1990s. *Home Healthcare Nurse* 8 (July/August):4.

CATCALL Collective (eds.). 1983. Feminist politics and women's health [Special issue]. *Catcall* 15:1–25.

CATCALL Collective (eds.). 1984. Feminist politics and women's health [Special issue]. *Catcall* 16:2–31.

Cayleff, Susan E. 1987. *Wash and be healed: The water-cure movement and women's health.* Philadelphia: Temple University Press.

Champlin, Leslie. 1991. Caring for older women: No more "hand-me-down" medicine. *Geriatrics* 46 (October):90–92.

Chavkin, W.; Cohen, J.; Ehrhardt, A. A.; Fullilove, M. T.; and Worth, D. 1991. Women and AIDS. *Science* 251 (January 25):359–360.

Childress, James F. 1982. *Who should decide? Paternalism in healthcare.* New York: Oxford.

Chin, J. 1990. Current and future dimensions of the HIV/AIDS pandemic in women and children. *Lancet* 336(8709):221–224.

Chu, Susan Y.; Buehler, James W.; and Berkelman, Ruth L. 1990. Impact of the human immunodeficiency virus epidemic on mortality in women of reproductive age, United States. *JAMA* 264(2):225–229.

Chu, Susan Y.; Buehler, James W.; Fleming, Patricia L.; and Berkelman, Ruth L. 1990. Epidemiology of reported cases of AIDS in lesbians, United States 1980–1989. *American Journal of Public Health* 80(11):1380–1381.

Claro, Amparo. 1991. Contraceptives from a woman's point of view. *ISIS Women's Health Journal* 1:4–9.

Cochran, Susan. 1990. Sex, lies, and HIV. *The New England Journal of Medicine* 322(11):774–775.

Cochran, Susan, and Mays, Vickie M. 1989. Women and AIDS-related concerns. *American Psychologist* 44(3):529–535.

Cochran, Susan D. 1989. Women and HIV infection: Issues in prevention and behavior change. In V. M. Mays, G. W. Albee, and S. F. Schneider (eds.), *Primary prevention of AIDS: Psychological approaches*, pp. 309–327. Newbury Park: Sage Publications.

Cohen, Nancy W., and Estner, Lois J. 1983. *Silent knife: Cesarean prevention and vaginal birth after cesarean.* South Hadley, Mass.: Bergin and Garvey.

Coney, Sandra. 1988. *The unfortunate experiment.* Auckland, New Zealand: Penguin Books.

Conley, Frances K. 1992. And ladies of the club (scientific societies and women's physicians. *JAMA* 267 (February 5):740–741.

Connors, Denise D. 1980. Sickness unto death: Medicine as mythic, necrophilic and iatrogenic. *Advances in Nursing Science* 2(3):39–51.

Cooke, M., and Ronalds, C. 1985. Women doctors in urban general practice: The patients. *British Medical Journal* 290:753–755.

Coombs, R. H., and Hovanessian, H. C. 1988. Stress in the role constellation of female resident physicians. *Journal of the American Medical Women's Association* 43:21–27.

Cope, Nancy R., and Hall, Howard R. (eds.). 1985. The health status of Black women in the United States [Special issue]. *Sage* 2 (Fall).

Corea, G.; Klein, R. D.; Hanmer, J.; Holmes, H. B.; Hoskins, B.; Kishwar, M.; Raymond, J.; Rowland, R.; and Steinbacher, R. (eds.). 1987. *Man-made women: How new reproductive technologies affect women.* Bloomington: Indiana University Press.

Corea, Gena. 1985. *The hidden malpractice: How American medicine mistreats women.* Updated ed. New York: Harper and Row.

Corea, Gena. 1992. *The invisible epidemic: The story of women and AIDS.* New York: Harper Collins.

Cotton, Paul. 1992. Women's health initiative leads way as research begins to fill gender gaps. *JAMA* 267 (January 22/29):467–470.

Cotton, Paul. 1992. Harassment hinders women's care and careers. *JAMA* 267 (February 12):778–779.

Coulter, Angela; McPherson, Klim; and Vessey, Martin. 1988. Do British women undergo too many or too few hysterectomies? *Social Science and Medicine* 27(9):987–994.

Culliton, Barbara J. 1991. NIH push for women's health. *Nature* 353 (October):383.

Dally, Ann G. 1991. *Women under the knife: A history of surgery.* New York: Routledge.

Dancy, Barbara L. 1991. The development of an ethnically sensitive and gender-specific AIDS questionnaire for African-American women. *Health Values: The Journal of Health Behavior, Education and Promotion* 15(6):49–54.

Davidson, Virginia. 1978. Coping styles of women medical students. *Journal of Medical Education* 53:902–907.

Davies, Celia. 1980. *Rewriting nursing history.* London: Croom Helm.

Day, Patricia. 1982. *Women doctors: Choice and constraints for medical manpower.* London: King's Fund Centre.

Dearing, R.; Gordon, H.; Sohner, D.; and Weidel, L. (eds.). 1987. *Marketing women's health care.* Rockville, Md.: Aspen Publishers.

de Bruyn, Maria. 1992. Women and AIDS in developing countries. *Social Science and Medicine* 34(3):249+.

Deevey, Sharon. 1990. Older lesbian women: An invisible minority. *Journal of Gerontological Nursing* 16(5):35–37, 39.

Delamont, Sara, and Duffin, Lorna. 1978. *The nineteenth-century woman: Her cultural and physical world.* London: Croom Helm.

del Portillo, Cerlotta T. 1987. Poverty, self-concept, and health: Experiences of Latinas. *Women and Health* 12(3/4):229–242.

Department of Health and Human Services. 1991. *Current issues in women's health.* DHSS Publication No. 91–1181. Rockville, Md.: Department of Health and Human Services, Public Health Service, Food and Drug Administration.

Dickson, Geri L. 1990. A feminist poststructuralist analysis of the knowledge of menopause. *Advances in Nursing Science* 12(3):15–31.

Dickstein, Leah J., and Nadelson, Carol C. (eds.). 1986. *Women physicians in leadership roles.* Washington, D.C.: American Psychiatric Press.

Doane, Mary Ann. 1985. The clinical eye. In S. Suleiman (ed.), *The Female Body in Western Culture*, pp. 152–174. Cambridge, Mass.: Harvard University Press.

Donegan, Jane B. 1986. *Hydropathic highway to health: Women and water-cure in antebellum America.* New York: Greenwood Press.

Donnison, Jean. 1977. *Midwives and medical men.* New York: Schocken Books.

Doyal, Lesley. 1983. Women, health, and the sexual division of labour: A case study of the women's health movement in Britain. *Critical Social Policy* 3(1):21–33.

Drachman, Virginia. 1982. Female solidarity and professional success: The dilemma of women doctors in late-nineteenth century America. *Journal of Social History* 15 (Summer):607–619.

Drachman, Virginia. 1984. *Hospital with a heart: Women doctors and the paradox of separatism at the New England Hospital, 1862–1969.* Ithaca: Cornell University Press.

Dreifus, Claudia. (ed.). 1977. *Seizing our bodies: The politics of women's health.* New York: Vintage.

Ducker, D. G. 1987. Life satisfactions for women physicians. *Journal of the American Medical Women's Association* 42:57–59.

Duden, Barbara. 1991. *The woman beneath the skin: A doctor's patients in eighteenth-century Germany.* Cambridge, Mass.: Harvard University Press.

Duffy, Mary E. 1985. A critique of research: A feminist perspective . . . male bias in research. *Health Care for Women International* 6(5/6):341–352.

Dumas, Linda. 1991. Women with AIDS. *Journal of Home Health Care Practice* 3 (May):11–23.

Dykman, R., and Stalnaker, J. 1957. Survey of women physicians graduating from medical schools, 1925–1940. *Journal of Medical Education* 32:3–38.

Edelman, Debra. 1986. University health services sponsoring lesbian health workshops: Implications and accessibility. *Journal of American College Health* 35(1):44–45.

Edemikpong, Ntiense Ben. 1990. Women and AIDS (in Africa). *Women and Therapy* 10(3):25–34.

Ehrenreich, Barbara, and English, Deirdre. 1972. *Witches, midwives and nurses: A history of women healers.* Old Westbury, N.Y.: Feminist Press.

Ehrenreich, Barbara, and English, Deirdre. 1973. *Complaints and disorders: The sexual politics of sickness.* Old Westbury, N.Y.: Feminist Press.

Ehrenreich, Barbara, and English, Deirdre. 1979. *For her own good: 150 years of the experts' advice to women.* London: Pluto Press.

Eichenbaum, Louise, and Orbach, Susie. 1983. *Understanding women: A feminist psychoanalytic approach.* New York: Basic.

Eisenberg, Carole. 1983. Women as physicians. *Journal of Medical Education* 58:534–541.

Eisenberg, Carole. 1989. Medicine is no longer a man's profession: Or when the men's club goes coed it's time to change the regs. *New England Journal of Medicine* 321 (November 30):1542–1544. Discussion, 323 (December 6, 1989):1637–1638.

Ellerock, T. V., and Rogers, M. F. 1990. Epidemiology of human immunodeficiency virus infection in women in the United States. *Obstetrics and Gynecology Clinics of North America* 17(3):523–543.

Ellison, P. T. 1990. Human ovarian function and reproductive ecology: New hypotheses. *American Anthropologist* 92 (December):933–952.

Elston, M. A. 1981. Medicine as old husbands' tales: The impact of feminism. In D. Spender (ed.), *Men's studies modified*, pp. 189–212. London: Pergamon.

Epps, Roselyn E. 1986. The Black woman physican: Perspectives and priorities. *Journal of the National Medical Association* 78(5):375–381.

Ettinger, Shelley. 1991. AIDS crisis is deadly for women. *New Directions for Women* 20 (March/April):12.

Eve, Susan B. 1988. A longitudinal study of use of health care services among older women. *Journal of Gerontology* 43(2):M31– M39.

Fausto-Sterling, Anne. 1986. *Myths of gender.* New York: Basic.

Fee, Elizabeth (ed.). 1983. *The politics of sex in medicine.* Farmingdale, N.Y.: Baywood.

Feldman, Douglas (ed.). 1990. *Cultural Aspects of AIDS.* New York: Praeger.

Felkner, M. 1982. The political economy of sexism in industrial health. *Social Science and Medicine* 16:3–13.

Femmes, Savoir, Sante (Women, Knowledge, Health—The whole issues). 1991. *Recherches Feministes* 4(1).

Field, P. A. 1990. Impressions of women's health in New Zealand. *Midwifery* 6(4):185–192.

Fisher, Anne. E. 1978. *Women's worlds: NIMH supported research on women.* DHEW Publication 78–660. Rockville, Md.: U.S. Government Printing Office.

Fisher, Sue. 1986. *In the patient's best interest: Women and the politics of medical decisions.* New Brunswick, N.J.: Rutgers University Press.

Flam, Faye. 1991. Women's health: A world crisis. *Science* 252 (June 21):1512.

Flam, Faye. 1991. House bill tells NIH to stress women. *Science* 253 (August 9):621.

Fletcher, Suzy. 1990. AIDS and women: An international perspective. *Health Care for Women International* 11 (Winter):33–42.

Foley, Mary Jo. 1990. Health research slights women. *New Directions for Women* 19 (November/December):4.

Foley, M. Jo, and Orloff, Tracy. 1987. Women and the politics of AIDS. *ISIS Women's World* 16 (December):8–9.

Fooden, Myra; Gordon, Susan; and Hughley, Betty (eds.). 1983. *The second X and women's health.* New York: Gordian Press.

Fullilove, Mindy T.; Fullilove, Robert E. II; Haynes, Katherine; and Gross, Shirley. 1990. Black women and AIDS prevention: A view towards understanding the gender rules. *The Journal of Sex Research* 27(1):47–64.

Gershon, Diane. 1992. Drug development: Drugs tested for women. *Nature* 355 (January 23):287.

Gillespie, Marcia A. 1991. HIV—The global crisis. *Ms.* 1 (January/February):17–22.

Giorgas, Belkis W. 1986. *A selected and annotated bibliography on women and health in Africa.* [Dakar, Senegal]: Association of African Women for Research and Development.

Goldsmith, Marsha F. 1990. Heart research efforts aim at fairness to women in terms of causes, care of cardiac disorders. *JAMA* 264 (December 26):3112–3113.

Goodman, Madeleine. 1980. Toward a biology of menopause. *Signs* 5(4):739–753.

Gordon, Linda. 1977. *Woman's body, woman's right: A social history of birth control in America.* New York: Grossman.

Gove, Walter R. 1984. Gender differences in mental and physical illness: The effects of fixed roles and nurturant roles. *Social Science and Medicine* 19:84.

Gradin, Anita. 1988. The power over medical research. *Women and Health* 13(3–4):175–180.

Grant, L. 1988. The gender climate of medical school. *Journal of the American Medical Women Association* 43:109–114.

Grau, Lois. 1987. Illness-engendered poverty among the elderly. *Women and Health* 12(3/4):103–118.

Gray, C. 1980. How will the new wave of women graduates change the medical profession? *Canadian Medical Association Journal* 123:798–804.

Greenberg, Dan. 1990. Where were all the women? *New Scientist* 128 (October 27):57.

Greer, S.; Dickerson, V.; and Schneiderman, L. J. 1986. Responses of male and female physicians to medical complaints in male and female patients. *Journal of Family Practice* 23(1):49–53.

Griffith-Kenney, Janet W. 1986. *Contemporary women's health: A nursing advocacy approach.* Menlo Park, Calif.: Addison-Wesley.

Guinan, Mary E., and Hardy, Ann. 1987. Epidemiology of AIDS in women in the United States. *Journal of the American Medical Women's Association* 257(15):2039–2042.

Haines, J. 1991. Women and AIDS. *Canadian Nurse* 87 (February):15–17.

Haller, John S. 1974. *The physician and sexuality in Victorian America.* Urbana: University of Illinois Press.

Hamilton, David P. 1991. NIH overwhelmed by response to women's health initiative. *Science* 252 (May 10):767.

Hamilton, J., and Harris, J. 1983. Sex-related differences in clinical drug response: Implications for women's health. *Journal of the American Medical Women's Association* 38(5):126–138.

Hammond, Doris B. 1986. Health care for older women: Curing the disease. *Women and Politics* 6 (Summer):59–69.

Harding, N. 1989. The use and abuse of women in the NHS. *Radical Community Medicine* 27:6–10.

Harris, J. 1984. Women in medicine: Making a difference in health policy. *JAMA* 39(3):77–79.

Harrison, Michelle. 1983. *A woman in residence: A doctor's personal and professional battles vs. an insensitive medical system.* New York: Random.

Hartmann, Betsy. 1987. *Reproductive rights and wrongs: The global politics of population control and contraceptive choice.* New York: Harper and Row.

Haug, Marie R., and Folmar, Steven J. 1986. Longevity, gender, and life quality. *Journal of Health and Social Behavior* 27 (December):332–345.

Haug, Marie R.; Ford, Amasa B.; and Sheafor, Marion (eds.). 1985. *The physical and mental health of aged women.* New York: Springer.

Healy, Bernadine. 1991. Women's health, public welfare. *JAMA* 266 (July 24/31):566–568.

Hedman, Birgitta, and Herner, E. 1988. Women's health and women's work in health services: What statistics tell us. *Women and Health* 13(3/4):9–34.

Heide, Wilma Scott. 1985. *Feminism for the health of it.* Buffalo, N.Y.: Margaret Daughters.

Heins, M. 1983. Medicine and motherhood. *JAMA* 249(2):209–210.

Heins, M.; Smack, S.; and Martindale, L. 1978. Current status of women physicians. *International Journal of Women's Studies* 1(3):297–305.

Heise, L. 1990. Crimes of gender. *Women's Health Journal* 17 (January–March):10.

Hepburn, Cuca, with Gutierrez, Bonnie. 1988. *Alive and well: A lesbian health guide.* Freedom, Calif.: Crossing.

Herzenberg, Caroline L.; Meschel, Susan V.; and Altena, James A. 1991. Women scientists and physicians of antiquity and the Middle Ages. *Journal of Chemical Education* 68 (February):101–105.

Hibbard, Judith H., and Pope, Clyde R. 1983. Gender roles, illness orientation and use of medical services. *Social Science and Medicine* 17(3):129–137.

Hine, Darlene Clark. 1989. *Black women in white: Racial conflict and cooperation in the nursing profession, 1890–1950.* Bloomington: Indiana University Press.

Hitchcock, Janice. 1989. Bibliography on lesbian health. *Women's Studies* 17(1/2):139+.

Holloway, Marguerite, and Yam, Philip. 1992. Reflecting differences: Health care begins to address needs of women and minorities. *Scientific American* 266 (March):13.

Holmes, Helen B., and Purdy, Laura M. (eds.). 1992. *Feminist perspectives in medical ethics.* Bloomington: Indiana University Press.

Hsia, Lily. 1991. Midwives and the empowerment of women: An international perspective. *Journal of Nurse Midwifery* 36:85–87.

Hubbard, Ruth. 1990. *The politics of women's biology.* New Brunswick: Rutgers University Press.

Hubbard, Ruth, and Henifin, Mary Sue (eds.). 1982. *Biological woman—The convenient myth: A collection of feminist essays and a comprehensive bibliography.* Cambridge, Mass.: Schenkman.

Hughes, Tonda L. 1990. Evaluating research on chemical dependency among women: A women's health perspective. *Family and Community Health* 13(3):35–46.

Hutter, Bridgett, and Williams, Gillian (eds.). 1981. *Controlling women: The normal and the deviant.* London: Croom and Helm.

Jacker, N. S. 1991. Age-based rationing and women. *JAMA* 266 (December 4):3012–3015. Discussion, *JAMA* 267 (March 25, 1992):1612–1613.

Jacobus, Mary; Keller, Evelyn Fox; and Shuttleworth, Sally (eds.). 1990. *Body/politics: Women and the discourses of science.* New York: Routledge.

Janus, L. 1983. Residents: The pressures on the women. *Journal of the American Medical Women's Association* 38:18–21.

Johnson, S. R.; Guenther, S. M.; Laube, D. W.; and Keettel, W. C. 1981. Factors influencing lesbian gynecologic care: A preliminary study. *American Journal of Obstetrics and Gynecology* 140(1):23.

Johnson, Susan R., and Guenther, Susan M. 1987. The role of "coming out" by the lesbians in the physician-patient relationship. [Special issue: Women, power, and therapy: Issues for women.] *Women and Therapy* 6(1–2):231–238.

Kahn, Ethel D. 1984. The women's movement and older women's health: Issues and policy implications. *Women and Health* 9(4):87–100.

Kane, J. B. 1989. Women as managers in the health services. *Curationis: South African Journal of Nursing* 12(1/2):5–8.

Kane, Penny. 1991. *Women's health from womb to tomb.* New York: St. Martin's.

Kaplan, Marcie. 1983. A woman's view of DSM-III. *American Psychologist* 38 (July):786–792.

Katz, Jay. 1984. *The silent world of doctor and patient.* New York: Free Press.

Kelly, Janis. 1988. The global impact of AIDS on women. *Off Our Backs* 18 (August/September):20–21.

Kenner, Charmian. 1985. *No time for women: Exploring women's health in the 1930s and today.* London: Pandora.

Kirschstein, Ruth L. 1991. Research on women's health. *American Journal of Public Health* 81 (March):291–293.

Klein, E. 1990. Speciality urged in women's health. *New Directions for Women* 19(1):1+.

Kletke, Phillip R.; Marder, William D.; and Silberger, Anne B. 1990. The growing proportion of female physicians: Implications for U.S. physician supply. *American Journal of Public Health* 80 (March):300–304.

Klimek, J. 1990. Infection control update: The 6th International Conference on AIDS 1990. *Asepsis: The Infection Control Forum* 12(2):12–18.

Koblinsky, Marjorie A. (ed.). 1993. *Health of women: A global perspective.* Boulder: Westview Press.

Koeske, Randi D. 1983. Lifting the curse of menstruation: Toward a feminist perspective on the menstrual cycle. *Women and Health* 8(2/3):1–16.

Krause, Paula S. 1989. Tears (intern weeps for dying three-year old and negative reaction of her instructors). *JAMA* 261 (June 23/30):3612.

Kutner, Nancy G., and Brogan, Donna. 1990. Gender roles, medical practice roles, and ob-gyn career choice—A longitudinal study. *Women and Health* 16(3–4):99–117.

Kutner, Nancy G., and Brogan, Donna. 1991. Sex stereotypes and health care—The case of treatment for kidney failure. *Sex Roles* 24 (March):279–290.

Laplatney, R. 1991. Women and AIDS: The evolution of an epidemic. *Journal of the New York State Nurses Association* 22 (June):18–23.

Laserman, J. 1981. *Men and women in medical school.* New York: Praeger.

Laws, Sophie. 1983. The sexual politics of premenstrual tension. *Women's Studies International Forum* 6(1):19–31.

Laws, Sophie. 1983. Women's health care and alternative medicine: Reasons to believe? *Catcall* 15:2–7.

Leavitt, Judith W. 1983. Science enters the birthing room: Obstetrics in America since the eighteenth century. *Journal of American History* 70 (September):281–304.

Leavitt, Judith W. 1986. *Brought to bed: Childbearing in America, 1750–1950.* New York: Oxford University Press.

Leavitt, Judith W. (ed.) 1984. *Women and health in America: Historical readings.* Madison, Wis.: University of Wisconsin Press.

Leeson, Joyce, and Gray, Judith. 1978. *Women and medicine.* London: Tavistock.

Legler, C. 1992. Who controls the practitioner-patient relationship? *Journal of the American Academy of Physician Assistants* 5(2):73–74.

Lesbians and AIDS: What's the connection? 1986. San Francisco: Women's AIDS Network of the San Francisco AIDS Foundation.

Levinson, Wendy; Tolle, Susan W.; and Lewis, Charles. 1989. Women in academic medicine: Combining career and family. *New England Journal of Medicine* 321 (November 30):1511–1517.

Lewin, Ellen, and Olsen, Virginia (eds.). 1985. *Women, health and healing: Toward a new perspective.* New York: Tavistock.

Lewis, Myrna. 1985. Older women and health: An overview. *Women and Health* 10(2/3):1–16.

Little, A. Brian. 1990. Why can't a woman be more like a man? *New England Journal of Medicine* 323 (October 11):1064–1065.

Lorber, Judith. 1984. *Women physicians: Careers, status, and power.* New York: Tavistock.

Loring, Marti, and Powell, Brian. 1988. Gender, race, and DSM-III: A study of the objectivitiy of psychiatric diagnostic behavior. *Journal of Health and Social Behavior* 29 (March):1–22.

Lovell, Mariann C. 1980. The politics of medical deception: Challenging the trajectory of history. *Advances in Nursing Science* 2(3):73–86.

Lowe, Marian, and Hubbard, Ruth (eds.). 1983. *Woman's nature: Rationalizations of inequality.* New York: Pergamon.

Makuc, Diane M.; Freid, Virginia M.; and Kleinman, Joel C. 1989. National trends in the use of preventive health care by women. *American Journal of Public Health* 79 (January):21–26.

Mandelbaum, Dorothy R. 1978. Women in medicine. *Signs* 4(1):136–145.

Mandelbaum, Dorothy R. 1981. *Work, marriage, and motherhood: The career persistence of female physicians.* New York: Praeger.

Mantell, J. E.; Schinke, S. P.; and Akabas, S. H. 1988. Women and AIDS prevention. *Journal of Primary Prevention* 9(1–2):18–40.

Marieskind, Helen I. 1980. *Women in the health system: Patients, providers, and programs.* St. Louis: C. V. Mosby.

Marieskind, Helen I. 1984. Research in women's health: Problems and prospects. *Journal of the American Medical Women's Association* 39:91–96.

Marshall, Eliot. 1990. Third strike for NCI (National Cancer Institute) breast cancer study. *Science* 250 (December 14):1503–1504.

Marte, C., and Anastos, K. 1990. Women—The missing persons in the AIDS epidemic. Part II. *Health/PAC Bulletin* (Spring):11–18.

Martin, Emily. 1987. *The woman in the body: A cultural analysis of reproduction.* Boston: Beacon.

Mason, James O. 1992. A national agenda for women's health. *JAMA* 267 (January 22/29):482.

Mason, Marion. 1987. Do you have any daughters: An update on the state of affairs between women scientists and the National Insitutes of Health. *Journal of the American Dietetic Associaton* 87 (March):283–284.

Matheson, Clare. 1989. *Fate cries enough.* Auckland, New Zealand: Sceptre.

Mathews, Joan J., and Zadak, Kathleen. 1991. The alternative birth movement in the United States: History and current status. *Women and Health* 17(1):39–56.

Mays, Vickie M., and Cochran, Susan D. 1987. Acquired immunodeficiency syndrome and Black Americans: Special psychosocial issues. *Public Health Reports* 102(2):224–231.

Mays, Vickie M., and Cochran, Susan D. 1988. Issues in the perception of AIDS risk and risk reduction activities by Black and Hispanic/Latina women. *American Psychologist* 43(11):949–957.

McBride, Angela B. 1987. Developing a women's mental health research agenda. *Image: Journal of Nursing Scholarship* 19(1):4–8.

Mendelsohn, Robert S. 1981. *Mal(e)practice: How doctors manipulate women.* Chicago: Contemporary Books.

Micale, Mark S. 1989. Hysteria and its historiography: A review of past and present writings (II). *History of Science* 27(78):319–351.

Miles, Agnes. 1988. *The neurotic woman: The role of gender in psychiatric illness.* New York: New York University Press.

Miller, Carol A. 1990. Women's health: A focus for the 1990s. *Bioscience* 40 (December):817.

Mindel, Charles H., and Kail, Barbara L. 1989. Issues in research on the older woman of color. *Journal of Drug Issues* 19(2):191–206.

Minkoff, Howard L. 1987. Care of pregnant women infected with human immunodeficiency virus. *JAMA* 258(19):2712–2717.

Minkoff, Howard L., and DeHovitz, Jack. 1991. Care of women infected with the human immunodeficiency virus. *JAMA* 266(16):2253–2258.

Mitchell, J. L. 1988. Women, AIDS, and public policy. *AIDS and Public Policy Journal* 3(2):50–52.

Mitchinson, Wendy. 1991. *The nature of their bodies: Women and their doctors in Victorian Canada.* Toronto: University of Toronto Press.

Moldow, Gloria. 1987. *Women doctors in gilded-age Washington: Race, gender, and professionalization.* Urbana: University of Illinois Press.

Moloney, J. 1989. Women's health: A socio-political perspective. *Nursing Praxis in New Zealand* 4(2):9–12.

Moore, Francis D., and Priehe, Cedric. 1991. Board-certified physicians in the United States, 1981–1986. *New England Journal of Medicine* 324 (February). Discussion, 325 (July 4, 1991):67–68.

Morantz, Regina; Pomerleau, Cynthia S.; and Fenichel, Carol H. (eds.). 1982. *In her own words: Oral histories of women physicians.* Westport, Conn.: Greenwood.

Morantz-Sanchez, R. M., and Zschoche, S. 1980. Professionalism, feminism, and gender roles: A comparative study of nineteenth-century medical therapeutics. *Journal of American History* 67 (December):568–588.

Morantz-Sanchez, Regina M. 1974. The lady and her physician. In M. S. Hartman and L. W. Banner (eds.), *Clio's consciousness raised: New perspectives on the history of women,* pp. 38–54. New York: Harper Torchbooks.

Morantz-Sanchez, Regina M. 1977. Making women modern: Middle class women and health reform in 19th century America. *Journal of Social History* 10 (Summer):490–507.

Morantz-Sanchez, Regina M. 1977. Nineteenth century health reform and women: A program of self-help. In G. B. Risse, R. L. Numbers, and J. W. Leavitt (eds.),

Medicine without doctors: Home health care in American history, pp. 73–93. New York: Science History Publications.

Morantz-Sanchez, Regina M. 1985. *Sympathy and science: Women physicians in American medicine.* New York: Oxford University Press.

Morgan, Elizabeth. 1980. *The making of a woman surgeon.* New York: Putnam.

Morgan, Kathryn P. 1991. Women and the knife. *Hypatia* 6(3):25–53.

Morgen, Sandra. 1986. The dynamics of co-optation in feminist health clinic. *Social Science and Medicine* 23(2):201–210.

Moscucci, Ornella. 1990. *The science of woman: Gynaecology and gender in England, 1800–1929.* New York: Cambridge University Press.

Mowbray, Carol T. 1984. Case study: Women and the health care system—Patients or victims. *Women and Therapy* 3 (Fall/Winter):137–140.

Muller, Charlotte F. 1990. *Health care and gender.* New York: Russell Sage Foundation.

Mulligan, Joan E. 1983. Some effects of the women's health movement. *Topics in Clinical Nursing* 4(4):1–9.

Munro, Kathy. 1991. The aftermath of the cervical cancer inquiry in New Zealand: An antipodal aberration or universal struggle? *Issues in Reproductive and Genetic Engineering* 4(1):31–39.

Murphy-Lawless, Jo. 1988. Silencing of women in childbirth, or let's hear it from Bartholomew and boys. *Women's Studies International Forum* 11(4):293–298.

Murray, Jane L. 1990. Women and the future of family practice? *American Family Physician* 42 (August):360+.

Nadelson, Carol, and Notman, Malkah T. (eds.). 1982. *The woman patient.* 2 vols. New York: Plenum Press.

Nelson, Lawrence J., and Milliken, Nancy. 1988. Compelled medical treatment of pregnant women: Life, liberty, and law in conflict. *JAMA* 259 (February 19):1060–1066. Discussion, 260 (July 1, 1988):31–32. Discussion, 261 (March 24/31, 1989):1729–1730.

Nickerson, Katherine G.; Bennett, Nancy M.; and Estes, Dorothy. 1990. The status of women at one academic medical center: Breaking through the glass ceiling. *JAMA* 264 (October 10):1913–1917.

NIH addresses women's ills. 1990. *Science News* 138 (September 22):180.

Norwood, Christopher. 1987. *Advice for life: A woman's guide to AIDS.* New York: Pantheon.

Oakley, Ann. 1984. *The captured womb: A history of the medical care of pregnant women.* Oxford: Basil Blackwell.

Ogle, K. S.; Henry, R. C.; Durda, K.; and Zivick, J. D. 1986. Gender specific differences in family practice graduates. *Journal of Family Practice* 23(4):357–360.

Olesen, Virginia. 1986. Analyzing emergent issues in women's health: The case of toxic shock syndrome. *Health Care for Women International* 7(1–2):51–62.

Olesen, Virginia (ed.). 1975. *Women and health care: Research implications for a new era.* Washington, D.C.: GPO.

Orr, J. 1989. Women's health—The feminist contribution. *Health Visitor* 62(1):16.

Osborn, June E. 1988. AIDS: Politics and science. *New England Journal of Medicine* 318 (February 18):444–447.

Overall, Christine (ed.). 1989. *Future of human reproduction.* Toronto: Women's Press.

Padgett, Deborah. 1988. Aging minority women: Issues in research and health policy. *Women and Health* 14(3/4):213–225.

Palca, Joseph. 1990. Women left out at NIH. *Science* 248 (June 29):1601–1602. Discussion, *Science* 251 (January 11, 1991):159.

Palca, Joseph. 1990. NIH adjusts attitudes toward women. *Science* 249 (September 21):1374.

Palca, Joseph. 1991. NIH unveils plan for women's health project. *Science* 254 (November 8):792.

Pan American Health Organization. 1984. *Women, health, and development in the Americas: An annotated bibliography.* Washington, D.C.: Pan American Health Organization.

Parker, Alberta. 1986. Juggling health care technology and women's needs. In J. Zimmerman (ed.), *The technological woman: Interfacing with tomorrow,* pp. 239–244. New York: Praeger.

Patton, Cindy. 1985. *Sex and germs: The politics of AIDS.* Boston: South End Press.

Patton, Cindy. 1990. *Inventing AIDS.* New York: Routledge.

Perales, Cesar A., and Young, Lauren S. (eds.). 1988. *Too little, too late: Dealing with the health needs of women in poverty.* New York: Harrington.

Perrone, Bobbette; Stockel, H. Henrietta; and Krueger, Victoria (eds.). 1989. *Medicine women, curanderas, and women doctors.* Norman: University of Oklahoma Press.

PHS launches action plan on women's health issues. 1991. *Public Health Reports* 106 (July/August):469.

Picture of health for midlife and older women in America. 1988. *Women and Health* 14(3/4):53–74.

Plant, Judith (ed.). 1989. *Healing the wounds: The promise of ecofeminism.* Toronto: Between the Lines.

Posner, Judith. 1979. "It's all in your head": Feminist and medical models of menopause (strange bedfellows). *Sex Roles* 5:179–190.

Puentes, Markides C. 1992. Women and access to health care. *Social Science and Medicine* 35(4):619–626.

Rakusen, J. 1982. Feminism and the politics of health. *Medicine in Society* 8:17–25.

Ratcliff, Kathryn S. 1989. *Healing technology: Feminist perspectives.* Ann Arbor: University of Michigan Press.

Rathbone-McCuan, Elaine. 1985. Health needs and social policy: The health care of elderly women. *Women and Health* 10(2/3):17–27.

Raymond, Janice G. 1982. Medicine as patriarchal religion. *Journal of Medicine and Philosophy* 7:197–216.

Read, V. 1990. Women and AIDS. *Australian Nurses Journal* 20 (November):22–24.

Relman, Arnold S. 1980. Here come the women. *New England Journal of Medicine* 302(22):1252–1253.

Relman, Arnold S. 1989. The changing demography of the medical profession. *New England Journal of Medicine* 321 (November 30):1540–1542. Discussion, 322 (May 3, 1990):1316–1319.

Richardson, Diane. 1988. *Women and AIDS.* New York: Methuen.

Rieder, Ines, and Ruppelt, Patricia (eds.). 1988. *AIDS: The women.* San Francisco: Cleis.

Roberts, Helen 1985. *The patient patients: Women and their doctors.* London: Pandora.

Roberts, Helen (ed.). 1981. *Women, health, and reproduction.* London: Routledge and Kegan Paul.

Roberts, Helen (ed.). 1990. *Women's health counts.* New York: Routledge.

Roberts, Helen (ed.). 1991. *Women's health matters.* New York: Routledge.

Rodin, Judith, and Collins, Aila (eds.). 1991. *Women and new reproductive technologies: Medical, psychosocial, legal, and ethical dilemmas.* Hillsdale, N.J.: L. Erlbaum.

Rodin, Judith, and Ickovics, Jeanette R. 1990. Women's health: Review and research agenda as we approach the 21st century. *American Psychologist* 45(9):1018–1034.

Rodriguez-Trias, Helen. 1992. Women's health, women's lives, women's rights. *American Journal of Public Health* 82 (May):663–664.

Rogers, Paul G. 1987. Improving communication between women and health care providers. *Public Health Reports* 102 (supplement) (July/August):141–142.

Rome, Esther. 1986. Premenstrual syndrome (PMS) examined through a feminist lens. *Health Care for Women International* 7(1/2):145–151.

Root, M. Jean. 1987. Communication barriers between older women and physicians. *Public Health Reports* 102 (supplement) (July/August):152–155.

Rosser, Sue V. 1991. AIDS and women. *AIDS Education and Prevention* 3(3):230–240.

Rosser, Sue V. (ed.) 1988. *Feminism within the science and health care professions: Overcoming resistance.* New York: Pergamon Press.

Rossi, Alice S. 1980. Life-span theories and women's lives. *Signs* 6(1):4–32.

Roter, Debra; Lipkin, Mack; and Korsgaard, Audrey. 1991. Sex differences in patients' and physicians' communication during primary care medical visits. *Medical Care* 29(11):1083–1093.

Ruzek, S.; Olesen, V.; and Clarke, A. (eds.). 1986. *Syllabi set on women, health and health: Fourteen courses.* San Francisco: University of California.

Ruzek, Sheryl. 1978. *The women's health movement: Feminist alternatives to medical control.* New York: Praeger.

Ruzek, Sheryl. 1980. Medical response to women's health activities: Conflict, accommodation and co-optation. In J. A. Roth (ed.), *Research in the sociology of health care,* vol. 1 of *Professional control of health services and challenges to such control,* pp. 335–354. Greenwich, Conn.: JAI Press.

Ruzek, Sheryl. 1986. Feminist visions of health: An international perspective. In J. Mitchell and A. Oakley (eds.), *What is feminism: A reexamination,* pp. 184–207. New York: Pantheon.

Ruzek, Sheryl (ed.). 1986. *Minority women, health and healing in the U.S.: Selected bibliography and resources.* San Francisco: University of California.

Sandelowski, Margarete. 1981. *Women, health and choice.* Englewood Cliffs, N.J.: Prentice-Hall.

Sapiro, Virginia (ed.). 1985. *Women, biology, and public policy.* Beverly Hills: Sage Publications.

Schaller, Jane G. 1990. The advancement of women in academic medicine. *JAMA* 264 (October):1854–1855. Discussion, 265 (February 27, 1990):975–976.

Schumacher, Dorin. 1990. Hidden death—The sexual effects of hysterectomy. *Journal of Women and Aging* 2(2):49–66.

Scully, Diana. 1980. *Men who control women's health: The miseducation of obstetrician-gynecologists.* Boston: Houghton Mifflin.

Scully, Diana, and Bart Pauline. 1972. A funny thing happened on the way to the orifice: Women in gynecology textbooks. *American Journal of Sociology* 78:1045–1049.

Segawa, Shigeko. 1990. Clinical trials: It's still a man's world. *Nature* 345 (June 28):254. Discussion, *Nature* 347 (October 1990):418.

Selik, R. M.; Hardy, A. M.; and Curran, J. W. 1989. Epidemiology of AIDS and HIV infection in women in the United States. *Clinical Practice of Gynecology* 1:33–42.

Shallat, Lezak. 1990. Women and AIDS: The unprotected sex. *Women's Health Journal* 18 (April–June):25–51.

Shallat, Lezak. 1990. Take back the earth: Women, health and the environment. *Women's Health Journal* 20 (October–December):30- 47.

Shayne, Vivian, and Kaplan, Barbara. 1991. Double victims: Poor women and AIDS. *Women and Health* 17(1):21–37.

Sherwin, Susan. 1987. Concluding remarks: A feminist perspective—Issues raised at the conference on women's health issues. *Health Care for Women International* 8(4):293–304.

Sherwin, Susan. 1992. *No longer patient: Feminist ethics and healthcare.* Philadelphia: University of Temple Press.

Shorter, Edward. 1982. *A history of women's bodies.* New York: Basic Books.

Shorter, Edward. 1991. *Women's bodies: A social history of women's encounter with health, ill-health, and medicine.* New Brunswick, N.J.: Transaction Publishers.

Silberger, Anne B.; Marder, William D.; and Wilkie, R. J. 1987. Practice characteristics of male and female physicians. *Health Affairs* 6 (Winter):104–109.

Simmons, R.; Kay, B. J.; and Regan, C. 1983. Women's health groups: Alternatives to the health care system. *International Journal of Health Services* 13(4):619–634.

Sloane, Ethel. 1985. *Biology of women.* 2nd ed. New York: John Wiley and Sons.

Smeltzer, Suzanne C. 1992. Women and AIDS: Sociopolitical issues. *Nursing Outlook* 40(4):152–157.

Smith, C. 1983. Is alternative medicine necessarily better for women? *Catcall* 15:8–14.

Smith, John M. 1993. *Women and doctors: A physician's explosive account of women's medical treatment and mistreatment in America today.* New York: Dell.

Smith-Rosenberg, Carroll, and Rosenberg, Charles E. 1973. The female animal: Medical and biological views of woman and her role in nineteenth century America. *Journal of American History* 60 (September):332–356.

Smyke, Patricia. 1991. *Women and health.* London: Zed Books.

Sofaer, Shoshanna, and Abel, Emily. 1990. Older women's health and financial vulnerability—Implications of the Medicare benefit structure. *Women and Health* 16(3–4):47–67.

Sontag, Susan. 1978. *Illness as metaphor and AIDS.* New York: Farrar, Straus, and Giroux.

Sontag, Susan. 1989. *AIDS and its metaphors.* New York: Farrar, Straus, and Giroux.

Spallone, Patricia, and Steinberg, Deborah L. (eds.). 1987. *Made to order: The myth of reproductive and genetic progress.* New York: Pergamon.

Spitzack, Carole. 1990. *Confessing excess: Women and the politics of body reduction.* Albany: University of New York Press.

Sprecher, Lorrie. 1990. Women with AIDS: Dead but not disabled. *The Positive Woman: A Newsletter by, for, and about the HIV-Positive Woman* 1(2):4.

Stage, Sarah. 1979. *Female complaints: Lydia Pinkham and the business of women's medicine.* New York: Norton.

Stanworth, Michelle (ed.). 1987. *Reproductive technologies: Gender, motherhood and medicine.* Minneapolis: University of Minnesota Press.

Stein, Zena A. 1990. HIV prevention: The need for methods women can use. *American Journal of Public Health* 80:460–462.

Stellman, Jeanne Mager. 1977. *Women's work, women's health: Myths and realities.* New York: Pantheon.

Stemerding, B., and de Roba, C. 1991. Women and AIDS: The seventh international conference on AIDS. *Women's Global Network of Reproductive Rights Newsletter* 35 (April–June):33.

Stephens, P. C. 1988. Women and AIDS in the U.S. *New England Journal of Public Policy* 4(1):381–401.

Stern, Phyllis Noerager (ed.). 1986. *Women, health, and culture*. Washington, D.C.: Hemisphere.

Stevens, Patricia, and Hall, Joanne. 1990. Abusive health care interactions experienced by lesbians: A case of institutional violence in the treatment of women. *Response to the Victimization of Women and Children* 13(3):23–27.

Stevens, Patricia E., and Hall, Joanne M. 1988. Stigma in lesbian women: Identifiability, health beliefs and health care interactions. *Image: Journal of Nursing Scholarship* 20(2):69–73.

Taylor, K. 1986. The whole picture: Our health reflects our lives. In M. Adelman (ed.), *Long time passing: Lives of older lesbians*, pp. 219–235. Boston: Alyson.

Thomas, Patricia. 1987. AIDS agenda slights women. *Medical World News* (July 27):12–13.

Tobin, J. N.; Wassertheil-Smoller, S.; Wexler, J. P.; and Steingart, R. M. 1987. Sex bias in considering coronary bypass surgery. *Annals of Internal Medicine* 107 (July):19–25.

Todd, Alexandra D. 1989. *Intimate adversaries: Cultural conflicts between doctors and women patients*. Philadelphia: University of Pennsylvania.

Toffler, G. H.; Stone, P. H.; Muller, J. E.; and Willich, S. N. 1987. Effects of gender and race on prognosis after myocardial infarction: Adverse prognosis for women, particularly Black women. *Journal of American College Cardiology* 9(3):473–482.

Toubia, Nahid. 1991. Feminists and contraceptive research: The dialogue has started. *ISIS Women's Health Journal* 1:6–8.

Travis, Cheryl B. 1988. *Women and health psychology: Biomedical issues*. Hillsdale, N.J.: L. Erlbaum.

Trippet, Susan E., and Bain, Joyce. 1990. Preliminary study of lesbian health concerns. *Health Values, Health Behavior, Education, and Promotion* 14(6):30–36.

Tronto, Joan C. 1987. Beyond gender difference to a theory of care. *Signs* 12(4):644–655.

Ulin, Priscilla R. 1992. African women and AIDS: Negotiating behavioral change. *Social Science and Medicine* 34(1):63–73.

Ungerson, Clare. 1987. *Policy is personal: Sex, gender and informal care*. London: Tavistock.

U.S. is launching a 10-year study of women's health. 1991. *American Journal of Nursing* 91 (June):11.

Ussher, Jane. 1990. *The psychology of the female body*. London: Routledge, Chapman and Hall.

Vallely, Bernadette. 1991. Women, health and the environment. *Health Visitor* 64 (February):44–46.

Verbrugge, L. M., and Wingard, D. L. 1987. Sex differentials in health and mortality. *Women and Health* 12(2):103–145.

Verbrugge, Lois M. 1984. A health profile of older women with comparisons to older men. *Research on Aging* 6(3):291–322.

Verbrugge, Lois M. 1985. Gender and health: An update on hypotheses and evidence. *Journal of Health and Social Behavior* 26:156–182.

Verbrugge, Lois M. 1986. From sneeze to adieux: Stages of health for American men and women. *Social Science and Medicine* 22(11):1195–1212.

Verbrugge, Martha H. 1988. *Able-bodied womanhood: Personal health and social change in nineteenth-century Boston*. New York: Oxford University Press.

Vertinsky, Patricia A. 1986. God, science, and the marketplace: The bases for exercise prescriptions for females in nineteenth century North America. *Canadian Journal of the History of Sport* 17(1):38–45.

Vertinsky, Patricia A. 1990. *The eternally wounded woman: Woman, doctors, and exercise in the late nineteenth century.* New York: Manchester University Press.

Vliet, E. L. 1992. Women's health imperatives: The year 2000 and beyond—Excluding women from major research studies. *Journal of the American Academy of Physician Assistants* 5(4):235–238.

Wallace Helen M., and Giri, Kanti. 1990. *Health care of women and children in developing countries.* Oakland, Calif.: Third Party Publishing.

Wallace, J. I. 1988. Human immunodeficiency virus infection in women. *New York Medical Quarterly,* pp. 140–143.

Wallen, J.; Waitzkin, H.; and Stoeckle, J. D. 1979. Physician stereotypes about female health and illness: A study of patient's sex and the informative process during medical interviews. *Women and Health* 4(2):135–146.

Waller, Kathy. 1988. Women doctors for women patients? *British Journal of Medical Psychology* 6(2):125–135.

Walsh, Mary Roth. 1977. *"Doctors wanted: No women need apply": Sexual barriers in the medical profession, 1835–1975.* New Haven: Yale University Press.

Walters, Vivienne. 1991. Beyond medical and academic agendas—Lay perspectives and priorities. *Atlantis* 17 (Fall/Winter):28–35.

Ward, A. D. 1973. "The fashionable diseases": Women's complaints and their treatment in nineteenth century America. *Journal of Interdisciplinary History* 4(1):25–52.

A warm gesture (sexual harrassment of women physicians). 1992. *JAMA* 267 (February 5):743.

Warren, Virginia. 1989. Feminist directions in medical ethics. *Hypatia* 4 (Summer):73–87.

Webb, Christine (ed.). 1986. *Feminist practice in women's health care.* Chichester, England: John Wiley.

Weilepp, Anne E. 1992. Female mentors in short supply. *JAMA* 267 (February 5):739+.

Weisman, Carol S. 1987. Communication between women and their health care providers: Research findings and unanswered questions. *Public Health Reports* 102 (Supplement) (July/August):147–151.

Weisman, Carol S., and Teitelbaum, Martha A. 1985. Physician gender and physician-patient relationship: Recent evidence and relevant questions. *Social Sciences and Medicine* 20(11):1119–1127.

Weiss, Kay (ed.). 1984. *Women's health care: A guide to the alternative.* Reston, Va.: Reston Publishing.

Wertz, Richard W., and Wertz, Dorothy C. 1979. *Lying in: A history of childbirth in America.* New York: Free Press.

West, Candace. 1984. "When the doctor is a 'lady'": Power, status, and gender in physician-patient encounters. *Symbolic Interaction* 7(1):87–106.

Weston, Louise, and Ruggiero, Josephine. 1986. The popular approach to women's health issues: A content analysis of women's magazines in the 1970s. *Women and Health* 10(4):47–62.

Whelehan, Patricia. 1988. *Women and health: Cross-cultural perspectives.* South Hadley, Mass.: Bergin and Garvey.

White, Evelyn (ed.). 1990. *The Black women's health book: Speaking for ourselves.* Seattle: Seal Press.

Whyte, Judith. 1985. *Girl friendly schooling.* London: Methuen.

Wilson, Janet, and Leasure, Renee. 1991. Cruel and unusual punishment: The health care of women in prison. *Nurse Practitioner: American Journal of Primary Health Care* 16(2):32, 34, 36.

Windom, Robert F. 1987. The changing challenges of women's health for society and the health care system. *Public Health Reports* 102 (July/August):349.

Wofsy, Constance B. 1987. Human immunodeficiency virus infection in women. *JAMA* 257(15):2074–2076.

Women and AIDS. [Special issue.] 1988. *ISIS Women's World* 18 (June).

Women begin to make gains in medical politics. 1988. *American Family Physician* 37 (June):84.

Women's health: A national priority. 1992. *American Family Physician* 45 (May):2399+.

Women's health: Specialty provokes debate. 1990. *Nursing* 20 (June):9.

Wood, Ann Douglas. 1973. "The fashionable diseases": Women's complaints and their treatment in nineteenth-century America. *Journal of Interdisciplinary History* 4 (Summer):25–52.

World Health Organization. 1985. *Women, health, and development: A report.* Geneva: World Health Organization.

Worth, Dooley. 1990. Women at high risk of HIV infection: Behavioral, prevention, and intervention aspects. In D. Ostrow (ed.), *Behavioral aspects of AIDS and other sexually transmitted diseases,* pp. 101–119. New York: Plenum Press.

Yogev, Sara, and Harris, Sharon. 1983. Women physicians during residency years: Workload, work satisfaction, and self concept. *Social Science and Medicine* 17(12):837–841.

Zambrana, R. E.; Mogel, W.; and Scrimshaw, S. C. M. 1987. Gender and level of training differences in obstetricians' attitudes towards patients in childbirth. *Women and Health* 12(1):5–24.

Zambrana, Ruth E. 1987. A research agenda on issues affecting poor and minority women: A model for understanding their health needs. *Women and Health* 12(3/4):137–160.

Zita, Jacquelyn N. 1988. Premenstrual syndrome: Diseasing the female cycle. *Hypatia* 3(1):77–99.

Index

abortion, 55, 59–60
accidents, in elderly, 78
African-American feminism, 132–34
African-American women: breast cancer, 89, 90; drug abuse, 97; health concerns of, 90–91; lack of clinical research on, 87; lupus erythematosus, 89; sexually transmitted disease, 96–97; social origins of increased death rates, 95; teenage pregnancy, 91–92, 98; women's history, 103. *See also* African-American feminism
ageism, health care for elderly, 73, 74, 78, 80, 83, 191
AIDS: etiology and diagnosis of in women, 6; Hispanic community, 116; limited research in women, 10, 11, 107–108; underdiagnosis and inadequate treatment in women, 16, 19–27, 190; women of color, 91, 92
Alaska Native women, 87
Alcoholics Anonymous (AA), 109
alcoholism: elderly women, 76–77; lesbians, 108–109; Native American women, 91, 97; sexism in psychiatry, 43; underdiagnosis in women, 39
American Medical Women's Association (AMWA), 157
American Psychiatric Association, 36, 37
American Psychological Association, 42
amniocentesis, 64, 66
Anastos, K., 21–22
androcentrism: in AIDS research, 19–27; elderly women and health care, 73–83; health care and bias in research, 190–91; in obstetrics/gynecology, 50–66; overview of bias in clinical research, 3–12; in psychiatric diagnosis, 31–45; sources of in science research, 16–18. *See also* sexism
animal models, 128–29
anthropomorphism, 128
Aristotle, 3, 51
arthritis, 75
Asian-American women: genetic disorders, 96; health concerns of, 90–91; lactose intolerance, 90; racial diversity among, 87, 94
Association of American Medical Colleges (AAMC), 169–71
Avery, Byllye, 134
Ayanian, J. Z., 11

Beauvoir, Simone de, 136–37
Belenky, Mary F., 178–82
Belle, D., 42
Bickel, Janet, 168
biological determinism, 11

Biology and Gender Study Group, 52, 53
Birke, Lynda, 31
bladder infections, 79
Bleier, Ruth, 11, 31, 32–33, 33–34, 35, 184–85
Boston Women's Health Book Collective, 141
breast cancer, 56, 76, 90, 106–107
Brenner, Stephen, 180
Broverman, I. K., 38

Campbell, Margaret, 166
cancer, rates among Black women, 88. *See also* breast cancer; cervical cancer; endometrial cancer; uterine cancer
Centers for Disease Control (CDC), AIDS and, 20, 21, 26, 108
cervical cancer, 106, 111, 114
child abuse, 95
childbirth, 57–58, 63–64, 135–36
Chinese-American women, 89
Chodorow, Nancy, 138, 140
class: AIDS and, 25, 26–27; and cultural bias in psychiatry, 42; physicians and, 162–63
classism, in AIDS research, 26–27
Clinchy, Blythe M., 178–82
Clinton, Hillary Rodham, 125
Collins, Patricia Hill, 91
community, women physicians and, 171–72
compensatory history, 102–103
contraception, 54–55, 57, 93, 183
culture, definitions of health and disease, 96

depression, 41, 42
development, theories of, 51–54, 151, 184–85
diabetes, 75, 79
Diagnostic and Statistical Manual of Mental Disorders (DSM-III-R), 36, 37
Dinnerstein, Dorothy, 138, 140
DNA, models of, 17–18
domestic violence, 44, 92, 95
double-blind study, 128–29
Dowie, Mark, 183
drug abuse: in African-American women, 97; in elderly women, 77; and pregnancy, 92
drugs: AIDS research and women, 23–24; dosages for Asian/Pacific women, 96; dosages for elderly women, 82; exclusion of women from research and testing, 8–9, 60; psychiatry and overuse in women, 41; women of color and high-risk research, 93
dysmenorrhea, 7–8, 56

eating disorders, 56
economics: socioeconomic status of elderly

Sue V. Rosser is Director of Women's Studies at the University of South Carolina, where she is also Professor of Family and Preventive Medicine in the Medical School. Her books on women, science, and women's health include *Teaching Science and Health from a Feminist Perspective*, *Feminism within the Science and Health Care Professions: Overcoming Resistance*, *Female-Friendly Science*, and *Feminism and Biology: A Dynamic Interaction*.